Welcome to the **"Vegan Anti-Inflammatory Cookbook for Seniors: 110+ Vegan Recipes for Seniors to Naturally Reduce Inflammation and Promote Health."** This cookbook is designed to empower seniors with the tools and recipes needed to embrace a plant-based, anti-inflammatory diet. Our goal is to help you enhance your health, vitality, and enjoyment of life through delicious and nutritious meals.

Why This Cookbook?

As we age, our nutritional needs change, and managing inflammation becomes increasingly important for maintaining overall health and well-being. This cookbook provides a collection of simple, flavorful, and effective recipes that cater specifically to seniors, making it easy to incorporate anti-inflammatory foods into your daily routine.

What You'll Discover Inside:

- 110+ Vegan Recipes: Explore a diverse array of recipes, including breakfasts, lunches, dinners, snacks, and desserts, all designed to be both delicious and anti-inflammatory. Each recipe is plant-based, ensuring you get the benefits of nutrient-rich, whole foods.

- Health Benefits: Learn about the anti-inflammatory properties of various plant-based ingredients and how they can help reduce inflammation, support heart health, improve digestion, and boost your immune system.

- Easy-to-Follow Instructions: Each recipe includes clear, step-by-step instructions, making it simple for seniors of all cooking skill levels to prepare nutritious meals.

- Practical Tips: Gain valuable insights into meal planning, grocery shopping, and ingredient substitutions to make vegan, anti-inflammatory cooking a seamless and enjoyable part of your lifestyle.

Why Choose Anti-Inflammatory Foods?

- Reduce Pain and Discomfort: Anti-inflammatory foods can help alleviate chronic inflammation, which is often linked to conditions such as arthritis, cardiovascular diseases, and diabetes.

- Boost Overall Health: Incorporating these foods into your diet can lead to better overall health, including improved energy levels, enhanced mental clarity, and a stronger immune system.

- Natural and Wholesome: Focus on whole, unprocessed plant foods that not only taste great but also support your body's natural healing processes.

Let's Get Cooking!

Whether you're new to vegan cooking or a seasoned plant-based eater, the "Vegan Anti-Inflammatory Cookbook for Seniors" is your go-to resource for creating meals that are as nourishing as they are delicious. Embrace the simplicity and benefits of plant-based, anti-inflammatory eating, and discover how easy it can be to enhance your wellness with every bite.

Let's embark on this journey to vibrant health and culinary delight together!

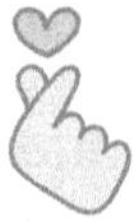

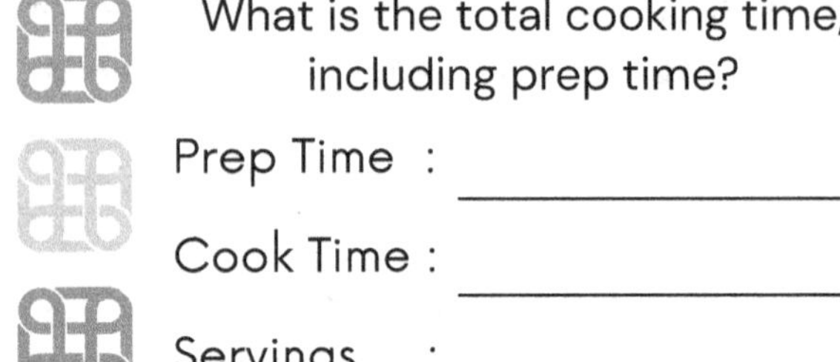

What is the total cooking time, including prep time?

Prep Time : _______________

Cook Time : _______________

Servings   : _______________

Ingredients:

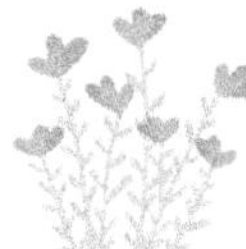

- 1 cup rolled oats
- 1 1/2 cups unsweetened almond milk (or milk of your choice)
- 1 tsp ground turmeric
- 1/2 tsp ground cinnamon
- 1 tbsp honey or maple syrup (optional)
- 1 cup fresh or frozen berries (such as blueberries, raspberries, or blackberries)

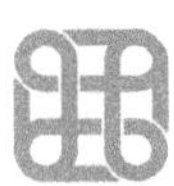
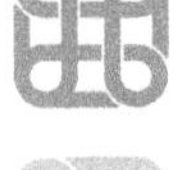
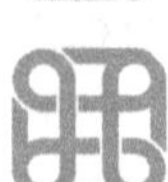
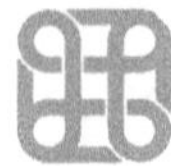

Is the recipe easy to follow?

1. Turmeric Oatmeal with Berries

1. In a medium saucepan, combine the rolled oats and almond milk. Bring to a simmer over medium heat, stirring occasionally.

2. Once the oats have thickened to your desired consistency, about 5-7 minutes, stir in the ground turmeric and cinnamon.

3. If desired, stir in the honey or maple syrup to sweeten the oatmeal.

4. Remove from heat and transfer the turmeric oatmeal to a bowl.

5. Top the oatmeal with the fresh or frozen berries.

6. Enjoy your warm, nourishing turmeric oatmeal with the sweet and tangy berries!

You can adjust the amounts of turmeric, cinnamon, and sweetener to your personal taste preferences. The turmeric adds a beautiful golden color and earthy flavor to the oatmeal.

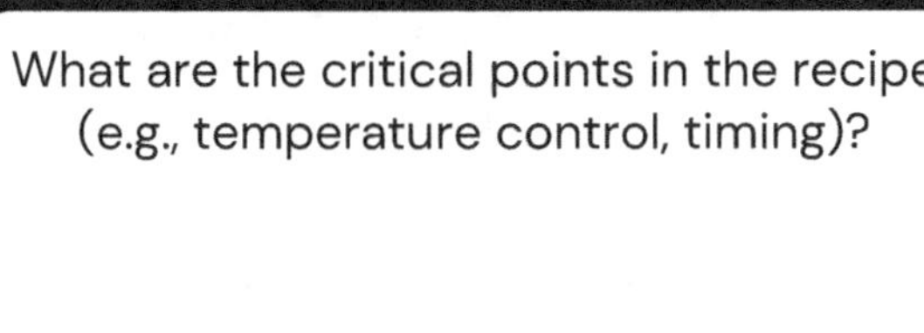

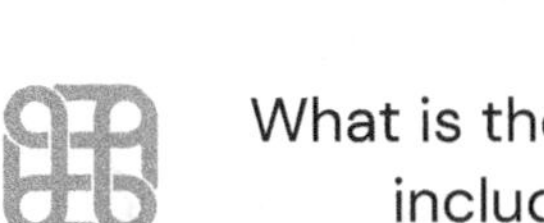

What is the total cooking time, including prep time?

Prep Time : ___________________

Cook Time : ___________________

Servings : ___________________

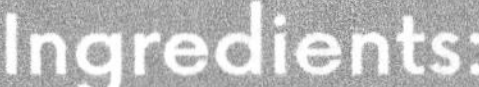 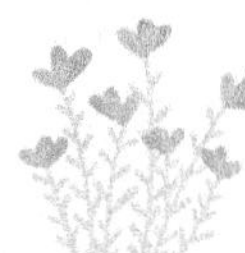

Ingredients:

- 1/4 cup chia seeds
- 1 cup unsweetened almond milk (or milk of your choice)
- 1 tbsp honey or maple syrup (optional)
- 1/2 tsp vanilla extract
- 1 cup fresh or frozen blueberries
- Ground cinnamon for topping (optional)

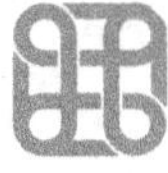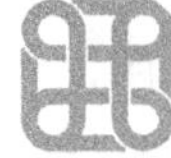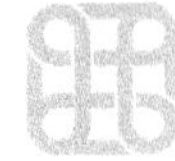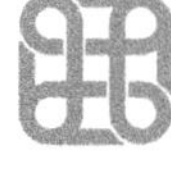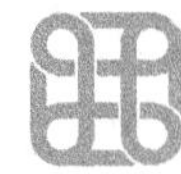

Is the recipe easy to follow?

2. Chia Seed Pudding with Blueberries

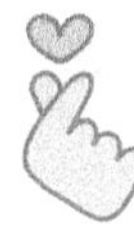

Procedure:

1. In a medium bowl, whisk together the chia seeds and almond milk until well combined.

2. Stir in the honey or maple syrup (if using) and vanilla extract.

3. Cover the bowl and refrigerate for at least 2 hours, or overnight, stirring occasionally, until the chia seeds have thickened the mixture into a pudding-like consistency.

4. When ready to serve, divide the chia seed pudding into individual bowls or cups.

5. Top each serving with a generous amount of fresh or frozen blueberries.

6. Optionally, sprinkle a dash of ground cinnamon over the top.

Why this is a great anti-inflammatory option for seniors:

- Chia seeds are high in omega-3 fatty acids, which have potent anti-inflammatory properties.
- Blueberries are rich in antioxidants and have been shown to reduce inflammation in the body.
- Cinnamon also has anti-inflammatory effects and can help regulate blood sugar levels.
- The overall nutrient-dense ingredients in this recipe can help support healthy aging and reduce inflammation in seniors.

This chia seed pudding is a simple, delicious, and nourishing breakfast or snack that can be enjoyed by people of all ages, especially seniors looking to maintain healthy inflammation levels.

What are the critical points in the recipe (e.g., temperature control, timing)?

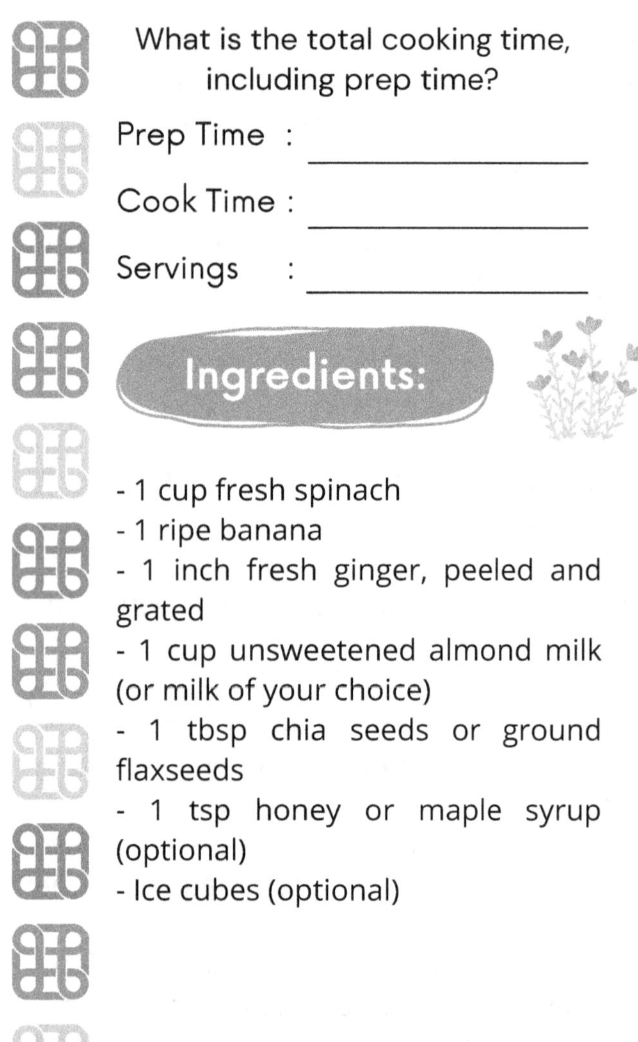

What is the total cooking time, including prep time?

Prep Time : ______________

Cook Time : ______________

Servings   : ______________

Ingredients:

- 1 cup fresh spinach
- 1 ripe banana
- 1 inch fresh ginger, peeled and grated
- 1 cup unsweetened almond milk (or milk of your choice)
- 1 tbsp chia seeds or ground flaxseeds
- 1 tsp honey or maple syrup (optional)
- Ice cubes (optional)

Is the recipe easy to follow?

3. Smoothie with Spinach, Banana, and Ginger

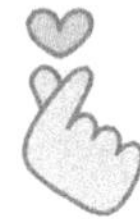

Procedure:

1. Add the spinach, banana, grated ginger, almond milk, chia/flaxseeds, and honey/maple syrup (if using) to a high-speed blender.

2. Blend on high speed until the mixture is smooth and creamy, about 1-2 minutes.

3. If you prefer a thicker, colder smoothie, add a few ice cubes and blend again briefly.

4. Pour the smoothie into a glass and enjoy immediately.

Why this is a great anti-inflammatory option for seniors:

- Spinach is rich in antioxidants and anti-inflammatory compounds like vitamin C, vitamin E, and carotenoids.
- Bananas are a good source of potassium, which can help reduce inflammation and blood pressure.
- Ginger is a powerful anti-inflammatory ingredient, known for its ability to reduce pain and swelling.
- Chia seeds and flaxseeds are high in omega-3 fatty acids, which have strong anti-inflammatory properties.

This smoothie provides a nutrient-dense, anti-inflammatory boost that can be especially beneficial for seniors. The combination of greens, fruit, and anti-inflammatory spices makes it a great choice for supporting overall health and reducing inflammation.

Remember, you can adjust the ingredients to suit your personal taste preferences. Enjoy this refreshing and nourishing smoothie as a healthy breakfast or snack.

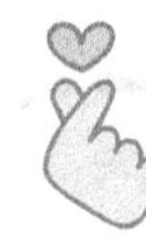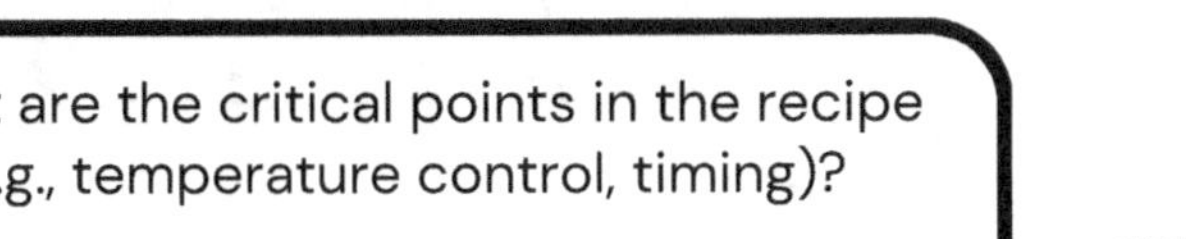

What are the critical points in the recipe (e.g., temperature control, timing)?

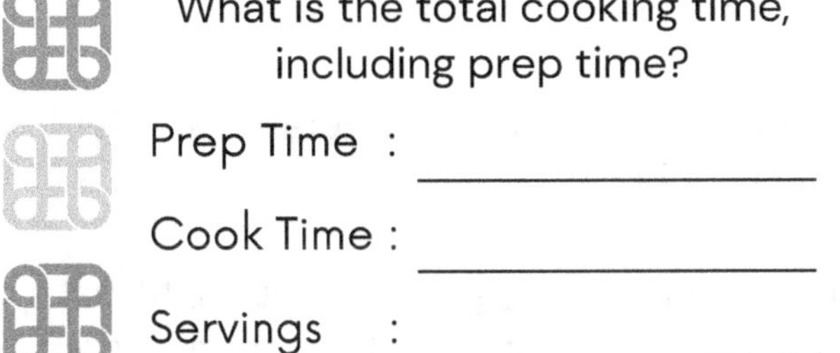

What is the total cooking time, including prep time?

Prep Time : ________________

Cook Time : ________________

Servings   : ________________

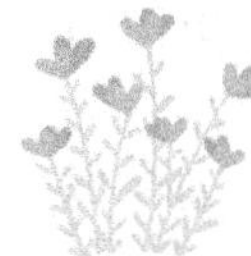

Ingredients:

- 2 slices of whole grain bread
- 1 ripe avocado, mashed
- 1 tbsp fresh lemon juice
- 1/4 tsp ground cumin
- 1/4 tsp ground turmeric
- 1/4 tsp garlic powder
- Salt and pepper to taste
- Optional toppings: sliced tomatoes, sprouts, crushed red pepper flakes

Is the recipe easy to follow?

4. Avocado Toast on Whole Grain Bread

1. Toast the whole grain bread until lightly golden.

2. In a small bowl, mash the avocado with a fork. Stir in the lemon juice, cumin, turmeric, garlic powder, salt, and pepper until well combined.

3. Spread the avocado mixture evenly over the toasted bread slices.

4. Optionally, top the avocado toast with sliced tomatoes, sprouts, or a sprinkle of crushed red pepper flakes.

Why this is a great anti-inflammatory option for seniors:

- Whole grain bread is a good source of fiber, which can help reduce inflammation in the body.
- Avocados are rich in healthy monounsaturated fats, as well as anti-inflammatory compounds like carotenoids and vitamin E.
- Lemon juice provides vitamin C, which has antioxidant and anti-inflammatory properties.
- Cumin and turmeric are both potent anti-inflammatory spices that can help reduce inflammation and pain.
- Garlic is also known for its anti-inflammatory effects, which can be beneficial for seniors.

This avocado toast is a simple, nutrient-dense, and delicious option that can help support healthy inflammation levels in seniors. The combination of whole grains, healthy fats, and anti-inflammatory ingredients makes it a great choice for a satisfying and nourishing meal or snack.

Remember to adjust the seasonings to your personal taste preferences. Enjoy this anti-inflammatory avocado toast!

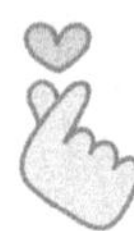

What is the total cooking time,
including prep time?

Prep Time : _______________

Cook Time : _______________

Servings   : _______________

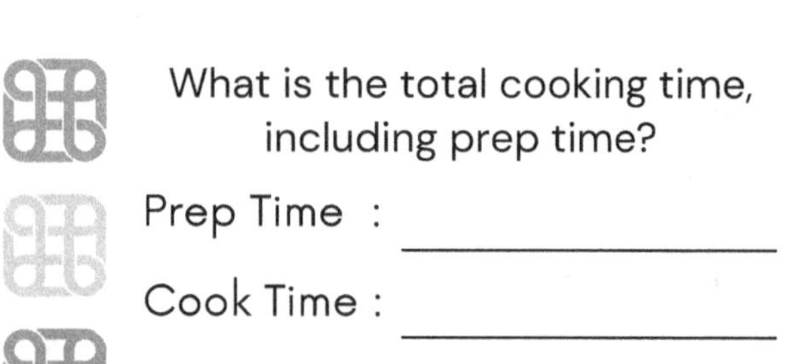

Ingredients:

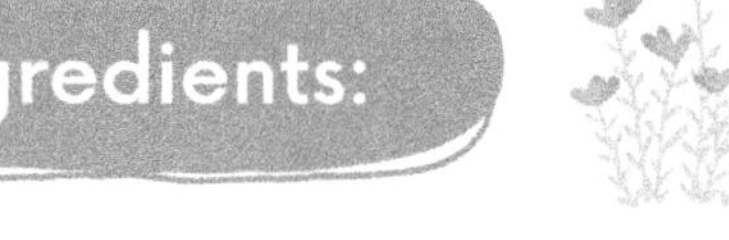

- 1/2 cup rolled oats
- 1 cup unsweetened almond milk (or milk of your choice)
- 1 tbsp almond butter
- 1 tbsp chia seeds
- 1 tsp honey or maple syrup (optional)
- 1/4 tsp ground cinnamon
- Pinch of salt

Is the recipe easy to follow?

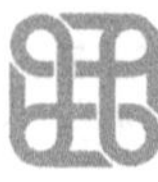 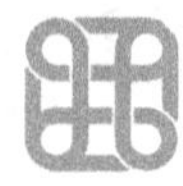  

5. Overnight Oats with Almond Butter and Chia Seeds

1. In a mason jar or airtight container, combine the rolled oats, almond milk, almond butter, chia seeds, honey/maple syrup (if using), cinnamon, and a pinch of salt.

2. Stir or shake the mixture until all the ingredients are well combined.

3. Cover the container and refrigerate overnight, or for at least 4 hours.

4. When ready to serve, give the overnight oats a stir and enjoy them chilled or at room temperature.

Why this is a great anti-inflammatory option for seniors:

- Rolled oats are a whole grain that is high in fiber, which can help reduce inflammation.
- Almond butter is a good source of healthy monounsaturated fats, which have anti-inflammatory properties.
- Chia seeds are rich in omega-3 fatty acids, which are known for their potent anti-inflammatory effects.
- Cinnamon is a spice with strong anti-inflammatory and antioxidant benefits.

This overnight oats recipe provides a nutrient-dense, anti-inflammatory breakfast or snack that can be especially beneficial for seniors. The combination of whole grains, healthy fats, and anti-inflammatory ingredients makes it a great choice for supporting overall health and reducing inflammation.

You can customize the recipe by adding other anti-inflammatory ingredients, such as berries, nuts, or a drizzle of honey or maple syrup. Enjoy this delicious and nourishing overnight oats dish!

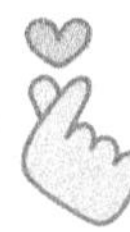

What are the critical points in the recipe (e.g., temperature control, timing)?

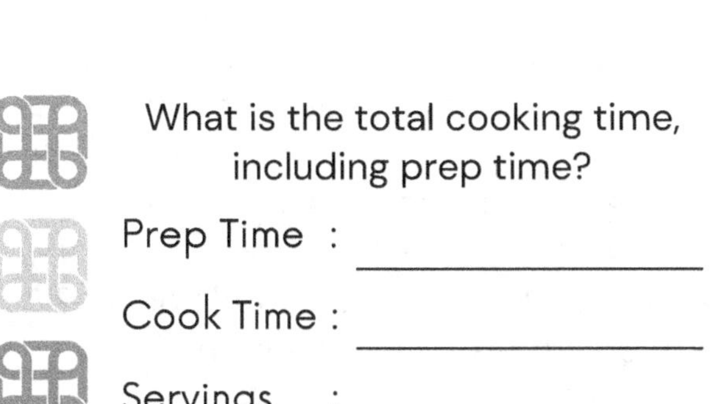

What is the total cooking time, including prep time?

Prep Time : _________________

Cook Time : _________________

Servings   : _________________

Ingredients:

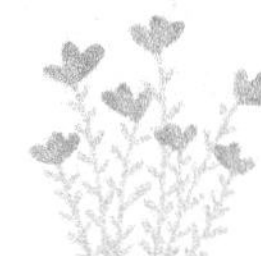

- 1 cup fresh kale, stems removed
- 1 cup frozen mango chunks
- 1 ripe banana
- 1 cup unsweetened almond milk (or milk of your choice)
- 1 tbsp chia seeds
- 1 tbsp ground flaxseeds
- 1 tsp honey or maple syrup (optional)
- Toppings: sliced almonds, shredded coconut, fresh berries

Is the recipe easy to follow?

6. Green Smoothie Bowl with Kale and Mango

1. In a high-speed blender, combine the kale, frozen mango, banana, almond milk, chia seeds, and flaxseeds.

2. Blend on high speed until the mixture is smooth and creamy, about 1-2 minutes.

3. If desired, add a teaspoon of honey or maple syrup to sweeten the smoothie.

4. Pour the blended smoothie into a bowl.

5. Top the smoothie bowl with your desired toppings, such as sliced almonds, shredded coconut, and fresh berries.

Why this is a great anti-inflammatory option for seniors:

- Kale is a nutrient-dense leafy green that is rich in antioxidants and anti-inflammatory compounds like vitamin C, vitamin K, and carotenoids.
- Mango is a tropical fruit that contains anti-inflammatory enzymes and vitamins, such as vitamin C and vitamin E.
- Bananas are a good source of potassium, which can help reduce inflammation and blood pressure.
- Chia seeds and flaxseeds are high in omega-3 fatty acids, which have strong anti-inflammatory properties.
- Almonds and coconut provide healthy fats that can also help reduce inflammation.

This green smoothie bowl is a delicious and nutrient-packed option that can support healthy inflammation levels in seniors. The combination of leafy greens, fruit, and anti-inflammatory ingredients makes it a great choice for a nourishing breakfast or snack.

What are the critical points in the recipe (e.g., temperature control, timing)?

What is the total cooking time, including prep time?

Prep Time : ___________________

Cook Time : ___________________

Servings   : ___________________

- 1 cup cooked quinoa
- 1 cup unsweetened almond milk (or milk of your choice)
- 1 medium apple, peeled, cored, and diced
- 1 tsp ground cinnamon
- 1 tbsp honey or maple syrup (optional)
- Pinch of salt

Toppings (optional):
- Chopped walnuts or pecans
- Sliced fresh apples
- Additional cinnamon

Is the recipe easy to follow?

7. Quinoa Porridge with Apples and Cinnamon

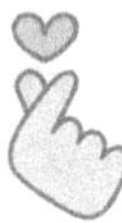

1. In a small saucepan, combine the cooked quinoa and almond milk. Bring the mixture to a gentle simmer over medium heat, stirring occasionally.

2. Once the quinoa porridge has thickened to your desired consistency, about 5-7 minutes, stir in the diced apple, cinnamon, honey/maple syrup (if using), and a pinch of salt.

3. Continue cooking for an additional 2-3 minutes, or until the apples are softened.

4. Remove the quinoa porridge from heat and transfer it to a bowl.

5. Top the porridge with your desired toppings, such as chopped walnuts or pecans, sliced fresh apples, and an extra sprinkle of cinnamon.

Why this is a great anti-inflammatory option for seniors:

- Quinoa is a whole grain that is high in fiber, protein, and anti-inflammatory nutrients like magnesium and B vitamins.
- Apples are a good source of antioxidants and anti-inflammatory compounds, such as quercetin and flavonoids.
- Cinnamon is a potent anti-inflammatory spice that can help reduce inflammation and pain.
- Walnuts and pecans are rich in omega-3 fatty acids, which have strong anti-inflammatory properties.

This quinoa porridge provides a nourishing, anti-inflammatory breakfast or snack that can be especially beneficial for seniors. The combination of whole grains, fruit, and anti-inflammatory ingredients makes it a great choice for supporting overall health and reducing inflammation.

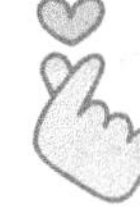

Procedure:

1. In a bowl or serving dish, place the unsweetened vegan yogurt.

2. Top the yogurt with the fresh berries, making sure to evenly distribute them.

3. Sprinkle the ground flaxseeds over the berries and yogurt.

4. If desired, drizzle a teaspoon of honey or maple syrup over the top for a touch of sweetness.

Why this is a great anti-inflammatory option for seniors:

- Vegan yogurt is a dairy-free, probiotic-rich option that can help support gut health and reduce inflammation.
- Berries, such as blueberries and raspberries, are packed with antioxidants and anti-inflammatory compounds like anthocyanins.
- Flaxseeds are a great source of omega-3 fatty acids, which have potent anti-inflammatory properties.
- Honey and maple syrup can provide a natural sweetener, while also offering some anti-inflammatory benefits.

This vegan yogurt parfait is a simple, yet nutrient-dense and anti-inflammatory option that can be enjoyed by seniors. The combination of probiotics, antioxidants, and anti-inflammatory ingredients makes it a great choice for supporting overall health and reducing inflammation.

You can experiment with different types of berries or other toppings, such as nuts or seeds, to customize the parfait to your liking. Enjoy this refreshing and nourishing vegan yogurt treat!

What is the total cooking time, including prep time?

Prep Time : _______________

Cook Time : _______________

Servings : _______________

Ingredients:

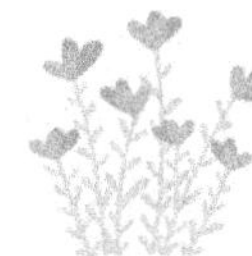

- 1 cup unsweetened vegan yogurt (such as coconut, almond, or soy-based)
- 1 cup fresh berries (such as blueberries, raspberries, or strawberries)
- 1 tbsp ground flaxseeds
- 1 tsp honey or maple syrup (optional)

Is the recipe easy to follow?

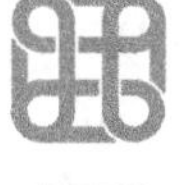
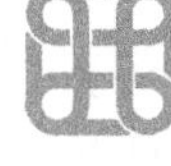
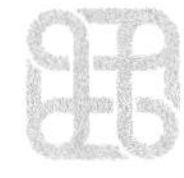
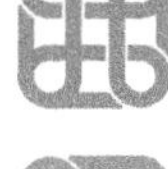
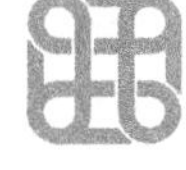

8. Vegan Yogurt with Fresh Berries and Flax Seeds

What are the critical points in the recipe (e.g., temperature control, timing)?

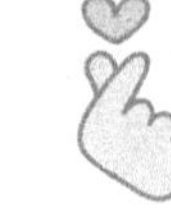

1. In a medium saucepan, combine the cubed sweet potato and almond milk. Bring the mixture to a simmer over medium heat.

2. Reduce the heat to low and let the sweet potato simmer, stirring occasionally, until it's very soft and the milk has thickened, about 15-20 minutes.

3. Remove the saucepan from the heat and mash the sweet potato with a fork or potato masher until it's smooth and creamy.

4. Stir in the ground cinnamon, ground ginger, and honey or maple syrup (if using). Add a pinch of salt to taste.

5. Transfer the sweet potato mixture to a bowl and top it with the chopped walnuts.

Why this is a great anti-inflammatory option for seniors:

- Sweet potatoes are rich in anti-inflammatory nutrients like vitamin A, vitamin C, and manganese.
- Cinnamon and ginger are both potent anti-inflammatory spices that can help reduce pain and swelling.
- Walnuts are a great source of omega-3 fatty acids, which have strong anti-inflammatory properties.
- The overall nutrient-dense ingredients in this recipe can help support healthy aging and reduce inflammation in seniors.

Feel free to adjust the sweetener and spices to your personal taste preferences. Enjoy this anti-inflammatory sweet potato breakfast bowl!

What is the total cooking time, including prep time?

Prep Time : ________________

Cook Time : ________________

Servings   : ________________

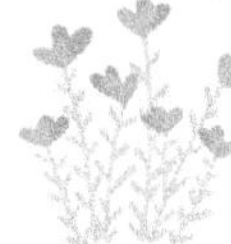

Ingredients:

- 1 medium sweet potato, peeled and cubed
- 1 cup unsweetened almond milk (or milk of your choice)
- 1 tsp ground cinnamon
- 1/4 tsp ground ginger
- 1 tbsp honey or maple syrup (optional)
- 2 tbsp chopped walnuts
- Pinch of salt

Is the recipe easy to follow?

9. Sweet Potato Breakfast Bowl with Walnuts

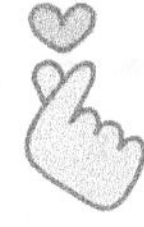

1. In a medium bowl, whisk together the buckwheat flour, baking powder, baking soda, and cinnamon.

2. In a separate bowl, whisk the almond milk, egg, and honey/maple syrup (if using) until well combined.

3. Pour the wet ingredients into the dry ingredients and stir just until the batter is smooth (do not overmix).

4. Heat a large non-stick skillet or griddle over medium heat and lightly grease it with coconut or avocado oil.

5. Scoop about 1/4 cup of the batter onto the hot skillet and cook for 2-3 minutes, or until bubbles start to form on the surface.

6. Flip the pancake and cook for an additional 1-2 minutes, or until golden brown.

7. Repeat with the remaining batter, greasing the skillet as needed.

8. Serve the buckwheat pancakes warm, topped with the fresh berries.

These buckwheat pancakes with fresh berries provide a delicious and nourishing breakfast or brunch option that can be especially beneficial for seniors looking to maintain healthy inflammation levels. The combination of whole grains, antioxidants, and anti-inflammatory ingredients makes it a great choice for supporting overall health.

Feel free to adjust the sweetener and toppings to your personal taste preferences. Enjoy these anti-inflammatory buckwheat pancakes!

What is the total cooking time, including prep time?

Prep Time : _______________

Cook Time : _______________

Servings : _______________

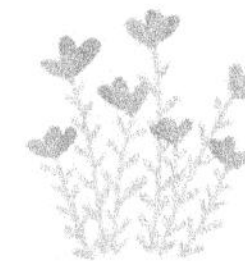

- 1 cup buckwheat flour
- 1 tsp baking powder
- 1/4 tsp baking soda
- 1/4 tsp ground cinnamon
- 1 cup unsweetened almond milk (or milk of your choice)
- 1 egg
- 1 tbsp honey or maple syrup (optional)
- 1 cup fresh berries (such as blueberries, raspberries, or a mix)
- Coconut oil or avocado oil for cooking

Is the recipe easy to follow?

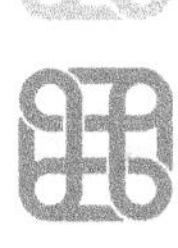

10. Buckwheat Pancakes with Fresh Berries

What are the critical points in the recipe (e.g., temperature control, timing)?

What is the total cooking time, including prep time?

Prep Time : ______________

Cook Time : ______________

Servings   : ______________

Ingredients:

- 2 medium carrots, peeled and cut into sticks
- 2 celery stalks, cut into sticks
- 1 cup homemade or store-bought hummus

Is the recipe easy to follow?

☺   ☹

11. Carrot and Celery Sticks with Hummus

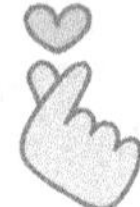

Procedure:

1. Wash and prepare the carrots and celery. Cut the carrots into long, thin sticks and the celery into 4-inch sticks.

2. Arrange the carrot and celery sticks on a serving platter or plate.

3. Place the hummus in a small bowl in the center of the platter, or serve it in a separate bowl alongside the vegetables.

That's it! This simple snack or appetizer is ready to enjoy.

Why this is a great option:

- Carrots are a great source of beta-carotene, an antioxidant that can help reduce inflammation.
- Celery is rich in vitamins and minerals, including vitamin K, which has anti-inflammatory properties.
- Hummus is made from chickpeas, which are a good source of plant-based protein, fiber, and anti-inflammatory compounds.

This combination of crunchy, nutrient-dense vegetables and protein-rich hummus makes for a satisfying and healthy snack. The antioxidants and anti-inflammatory properties of the ingredients can be especially beneficial for seniors.

You can customize this snack by using different types of vegetables, such as cucumber sticks or bell pepper slices. You can also experiment with different hummus flavors, such as roasted red pepper or garlic herb. Enjoy this simple, yet nourishing snack!

Procedure:

What is the total cooking time, including prep time?

Prep Time : ______________

Cook Time : ______________

Servings   : ______________

Ingredients:

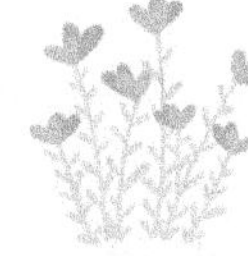

- 1 medium apple, cored and sliced
- 2 tablespoons almond butter
- Sprinkle of ground cinnamon (optional)

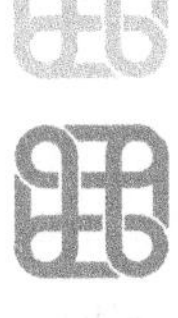
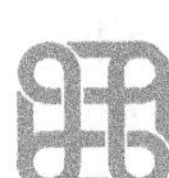
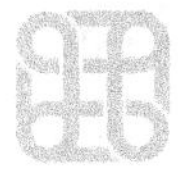
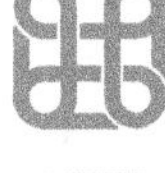
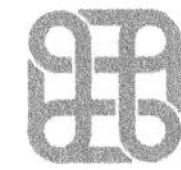

Is the recipe easy to follow?

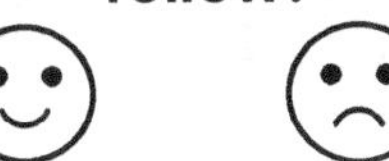

12. Apple Slices with Almond Butter

1. Wash and slice the apple into thin wedges or slices.

2. Spread a small amount of almond butter (about 1-2 teaspoons) onto each apple slice.

3. Optionally, sprinkle a light dusting of ground cinnamon over the almond butter-topped apple slices.

Why this is a great anti-inflammatory option for seniors:

- Apples are a good source of antioxidants and anti-inflammatory compounds, such as quercetin and flavonoids.
- Almond butter is rich in healthy monounsaturated fats, which have anti-inflammatory properties.
- Cinnamon is a potent anti-inflammatory spice that can help reduce inflammation and pain.

This simple snack provides a delicious and nourishing combination of anti-inflammatory ingredients that can be especially beneficial for seniors. The crisp, juicy apple paired with the creamy almond butter and the optional cinnamon topping creates a tasty and satisfying treat.

The healthy fats, antioxidants, and anti-inflammatory compounds in this snack can help support overall health and reduce inflammation in the body. It's a great option for a quick and easy snack or a light dessert.

Feel free to experiment with different types of apples or nut butters to find your favorite combination. Enjoy this anti-inflammatory apple and almond butter snack!

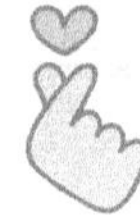

Procedure:

1. In a large bowl, combine all the ingredients - the almonds, walnuts, pecans, shredded coconut, dried cherries/cranberries, pumpkin seeds, ground flaxseeds, and ground cinnamon.

2. Stir the mixture well to evenly distribute all the ingredients.

3. Transfer the trail mix to an airtight container or resealable bag for storage.

Why this is a great anti-inflammatory option for seniors:

- Nuts like almonds, walnuts, and pecans are rich in healthy fats, antioxidants, and anti-inflammatory compounds.
- Dried cherries and cranberries are high in antioxidants and have anti-inflammatory properties.
- Pumpkin seeds are a good source of anti-inflammatory omega-3 fatty acids and zinc.
- Flaxseeds are packed with anti-inflammatory omega-3s and fiber.
- Cinnamon is a potent spice with strong anti-inflammatory effects.

This trail mix provides a nutrient-dense, anti-inflammatory snack that can be especially beneficial for seniors. The combination of nuts, seeds, dried fruits, and anti-inflammatory spices makes it a great choice for supporting overall health and reducing inflammation.

You can adjust the ratios of the ingredients to suit your taste preferences. Store the trail mix in an airtight container and enjoy it as a healthy snack throughout the day. It's a great option to have on hand for a quick and nourishing boost.

What is the total cooking time, including prep time?

Prep Time : _________________

Cook Time : _________________

Servings   : _________________

Ingredients:

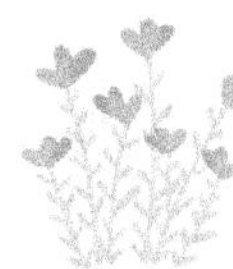

- 1/2 cup raw almonds
- 1/2 cup raw walnuts
- 1/2 cup raw pecans
- 1/4 cup unsweetened shredded coconut
- 1/4 cup dried cherries or cranberries
- 2 tbsp pumpkin seeds
- 1 tbsp ground flaxseeds
- 1 tsp ground cinnamon

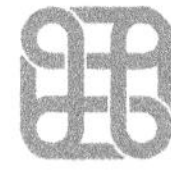
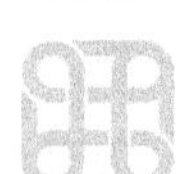
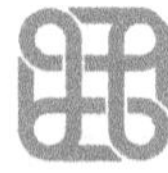
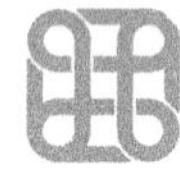

Is the recipe easy to follow?

13. Trail Mix with Nuts and Dried Fruits

What are the critical points in the recipe (e.g., temperature control, timing)?

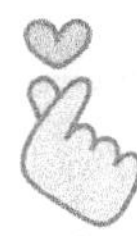

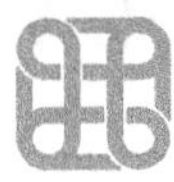
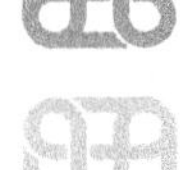

What is the total cooking time, including prep time?

Prep Time : ________________

Cook Time : ________________

Servings   : ________________

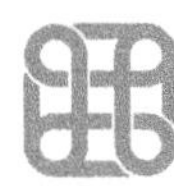

Ingredients:

- 1 large cucumber, sliced into rounds or half-moons
- 1 ripe avocado, mashed
- 1 tbsp fresh lime juice
- 2 tbsp diced red onion
- 1 tbsp chopped cilantro (or parsley)
- 1/2 tsp ground cumin
- 1/4 tsp garlic powder
- Salt and pepper to taste

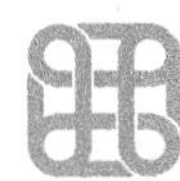

Is the recipe easy to follow?

14. Cucumber Slices with Guacamole

1. Wash and slice the cucumber into thin rounds or half-moons. Set aside.

2. In a small bowl, mash the avocado with a fork. Stir in the lime juice, diced red onion, chopped cilantro (or parsley), ground cumin, and garlic powder. Season with salt and pepper to taste.

3. Arrange the cucumber slices on a serving platter or plate.

4. Scoop a small amount of the guacamole onto each cucumber slice, spreading it evenly.

5. Serve the cucumber slices with guacamole immediately.

Why this is a great anti-inflammatory option for seniors:

- Cucumbers are hydrating and contain anti-inflammatory compounds like lignans and flavonoids.
- Avocados are rich in healthy monounsaturated fats, which have anti-inflammatory properties.
- Lime juice provides vitamin C, an antioxidant that can help reduce inflammation.
- Onions and garlic are both natural anti-inflammatory ingredients.
- Cumin is a spice with potent anti-inflammatory effects.

This cucumber and guacamole snack provides a refreshing, nutrient-dense, and anti-inflammatory option that can be especially beneficial for seniors. The combination of hydrating vegetables, healthy fats, and anti-inflammatory herbs and spices makes it a great choice for supporting overall health and reducing inflammation.

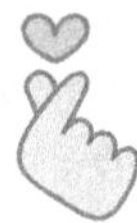

What is the total cooking time, including prep time?

Prep Time : _______________

Cook Time : _______________

Servings : _______________

Ingredients:

- 1 (15 oz) can of chickpeas, drained and rinsed
- 1 tbsp olive oil
- 1 tsp ground cumin
- 1 tsp ground turmeric
- 1/2 tsp garlic powder
- 1/2 tsp paprika
- 1/4 tsp cayenne pepper (optional)
- Salt and pepper to taste

Is the recipe easy to follow?

😊   ☹️

15. Roasted Chickpeas with Spices

1. Preheat your oven to 400°F (200°C).

2. Pat the drained and rinsed chickpeas dry with a paper towel or clean kitchen towel.

3. In a medium bowl, toss the chickpeas with the olive oil, cumin, turmeric, garlic powder, paprika, and cayenne pepper (if using). Season with salt and pepper to taste.

4. Spread the seasoned chickpeas in a single layer on a baking sheet lined with parchment paper.

5. Roast the chickpeas in the preheated oven for 20-25 minutes, stirring halfway, until they are crispy and golden brown.

6. Remove the roasted chickpeas from the oven and let them cool slightly before serving.

Why this is a great anti-inflammatory option for seniors:

- Chickpeas are a good source of plant-based protein, fiber, and anti-inflammatory compounds like folate and magnesium.
- Cumin and turmeric are both potent anti-inflammatory spices that can help reduce inflammation and pain.
- Garlic and paprika also have anti-inflammatory properties that can benefit seniors.
- The overall nutrient-dense and anti-inflammatory ingredients in this recipe make it a great snack choice for supporting healthy aging.

These roasted chickpeas with spices provide a crunchy, flavorful, and nourishing snack that can be especially beneficial for seniors. The combination of protein, fiber, and anti-inflammatory spices makes it a great option for supporting overall health and reducing inflammation

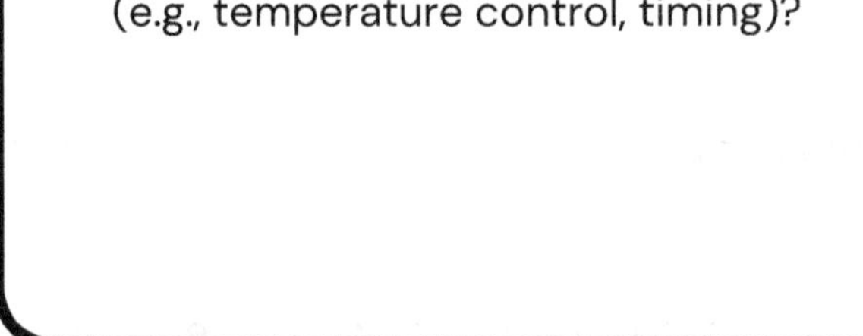

What are the critical points in the recipe (e.g., temperature control, timing)?

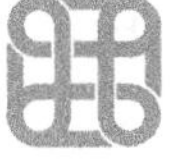

What is the total cooking time, including prep time?

Prep Time : _______________

Cook Time : _______________

Servings : _______________

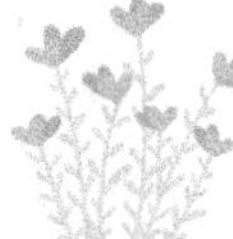

Ingredients:

- 1 cup raw almonds
- 1/2 cup raw walnuts
- 1/2 cup dried cranberries or blueberries
- 1/4 cup ground flaxseeds
- 2 tbsp honey or maple syrup
- 1 tsp ground cinnamon
- Pinch of salt

Is the recipe easy to follow?

16. Berry and Nut Energy Bites

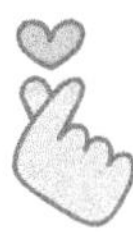

Procedure:

1. In a food processor, pulse the almonds and walnuts until they are finely chopped, but not turned into a butter.

2. Transfer the chopped nuts to a medium bowl and stir in the dried cranberries or blueberries, ground flaxseeds, honey or maple syrup, cinnamon, and a pinch of salt.

3. Using your hands, roll the mixture into small, bite-sized balls, about 1-inch in diameter.

4. Place the energy bites on a parchment-lined baking sheet and refrigerate for at least 30 minutes to help them firm up.

5. Store the energy bites in an airtight container in the refrigerator for up to 1 week.

Why this is a great anti-inflammatory option for seniors:

- Almonds and walnuts are rich in healthy fats, antioxidants, and anti-inflammatory compounds.
- Dried berries, such as cranberries and blueberries, are high in antioxidants and have anti-inflammatory properties.
- Flaxseeds are a great source of anti-inflammatory omega-3 fatty acids.
- Cinnamon is a potent spice with strong anti-inflammatory effects.
- The overall nutrient-dense and anti-inflammatory ingredients in this recipe make it a great snack choice for supporting healthy aging and reducing inflammation in seniors.

These berry and nut energy bites provide a convenient, portable, and nourishing snack that can be especially beneficial for seniors. The combination of healthy fats, antioxidants, and anti-inflammatory compounds makes it a great option for supporting overall health and reducing inflammation.

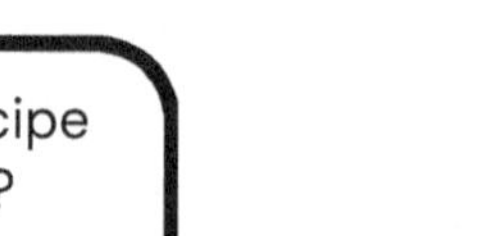

What are the critical points in the recipe (e.g., temperature control, timing)?

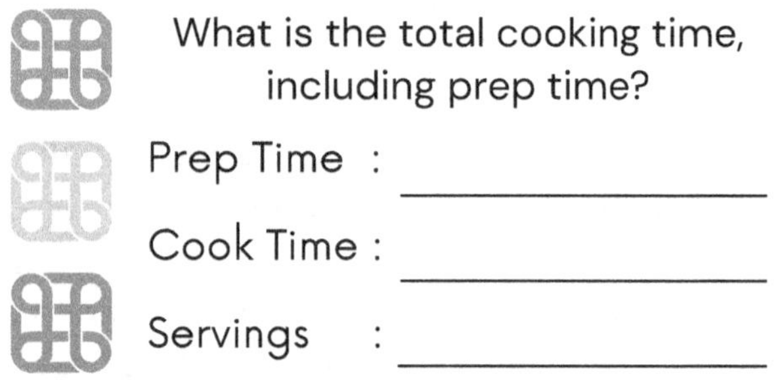

What is the total cooking time, including prep time?

Prep Time : _______________

Cook Time : _______________

Servings   : _______________

Ingredients:

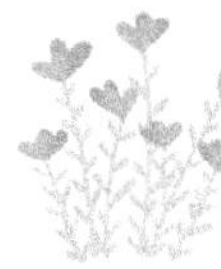

- 2 whole grain rice cakes
- 1 ripe avocado, mashed
- 1/2 cup cherry tomatoes, halved
- 1 tbsp fresh lemon juice
- 1/4 tsp garlic powder
- Salt and pepper to taste

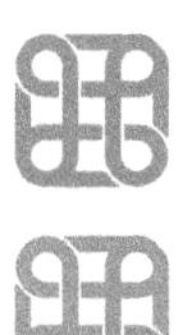
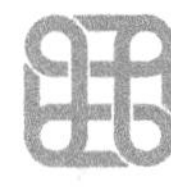
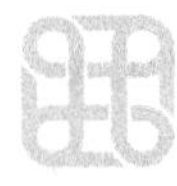
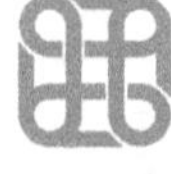
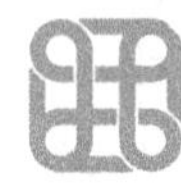

Is the recipe easy to follow?

17. Rice Cakes with Avocado and Cherry Tomatoes

1. In a small bowl, mash the avocado with a fork until it's creamy.

2. Stir in the lemon juice, garlic powder, and a pinch of salt and pepper.

3. Spread the mashed avocado evenly over the two rice cakes.

4. Top the avocado with the halved cherry tomatoes, arranging them in a decorative pattern if desired.

5. Serve the rice cakes immediately or refrigerate until ready to enjoy.

Why this is a great option:

- Whole grain rice cakes provide a crunchy, nutrient-dense base for the toppings.
- Avocado is rich in healthy monounsaturated fats, which can help reduce inflammation.
- Cherry tomatoes are a good source of antioxidants, such as lycopene, that have anti-inflammatory properties.
- Lemon juice adds a refreshing, tangy flavor and provides vitamin C, an antioxidant.
- Garlic powder adds a savory depth of flavor and has its own anti-inflammatory benefits.

This simple, open-faced sandwich is a nutritious and satisfying snack or light meal. The combination of the creamy avocado, juicy tomatoes, and crunchy rice cakes creates a delightful texture and flavor profile.

This recipe is easy to prepare and can be customized to individual preferences. Feel free to experiment with different toppings or seasonings to suit your taste. Enjoy this healthy and flavorful rice cake creation!

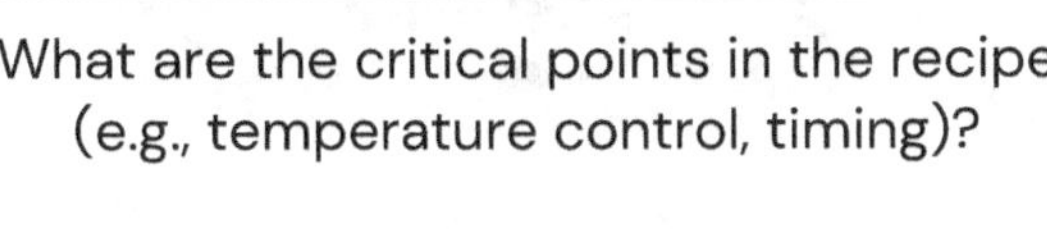

What are the critical points in the recipe (e.g., temperature control, timing)?

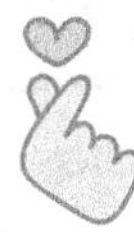

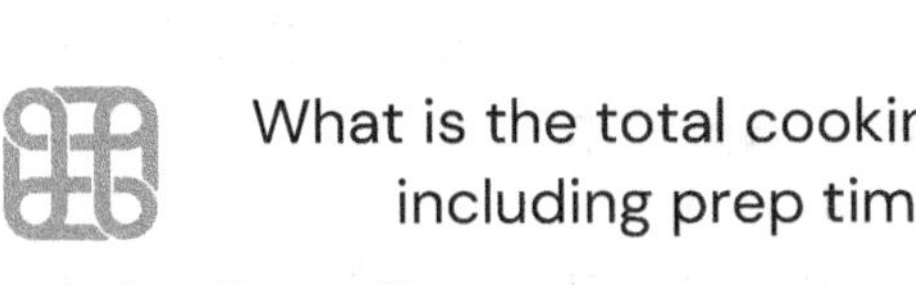

What is the total cooking time, including prep time?

Prep Time : ________________

Cook Time : ________________

Servings   : ________________

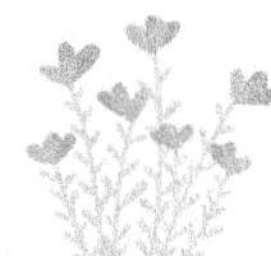

Ingredients:

- 1 cup diced pineapple
- 1 cup diced mango
- 1 cup halved strawberries
- 1 cup blueberries
- 1 cup diced kiwi
- 2 tbsp freshly squeezed lemon juice
- 1 tsp honey (optional)

Is the recipe easy to follow?

18. *Fresh Fruit Salad with Lemon Juice*

1. In a large bowl, combine the diced pineapple, mango, strawberries, blueberries, and kiwi.

2. Drizzle the freshly squeezed lemon juice over the fruit and gently toss to coat.

3. If desired, add a teaspoon of honey and toss again to lightly sweeten the fruit salad.

4. Serve the fresh fruit salad chilled or at room temperature.

Why this is a great anti-inflammatory option for seniors:

- Pineapple contains the enzyme bromelain, which has potent anti-inflammatory properties.
- Mangoes are rich in vitamins C and E, as well as antioxidants that can help reduce inflammation.
- Strawberries and blueberries are packed with anthocyanins, which are powerful anti-inflammatory compounds.
- Kiwi is a good source of vitamin C, an antioxidant that can help fight inflammation.
- Lemon juice provides additional vitamin C and can help enhance the absorption of the fruit's antioxidants.

This fresh fruit salad is a delicious and nourishing way to incorporate a variety of anti-inflammatory fruits into the diet. The combination of different fruits provides a range of vitamins, minerals, and antioxidants that can be especially beneficial for seniors.

You can adjust the fruit selection based on personal preferences or seasonal availability. The lemon juice helps to brighten the flavors and provide an extra anti-inflammatory boost. Enjoy this refreshing and anti-inflammatory fruit salad as a healthy snack or dessert.

What are the critical points in the recipe (e.g., temperature control, timing)?

What is the total cooking time, including prep time?

Prep Time : ___________________

Cook Time : ___________________

Servings : ___________________

Ingredients:

- 1 red bell pepper, sliced into strips
- 1 yellow bell pepper, sliced into strips
- 1/2 cup tahini
- 2 tbsp freshly squeezed lemon juice
- 2 tbsp water
- 1 garlic clove, minced
- 1 tsp ground cumin
- 1/4 tsp cayenne pepper (optional)
- Salt and pepper to taste

Is the recipe easy to follow?

19. *Sliced Bell Peppers with Tahini Dip*

1. In a medium bowl, whisk together the tahini, lemon juice, water, minced garlic, cumin, and cayenne pepper (if using). Season with salt and pepper to taste.

2. Arrange the sliced red and yellow bell pepper strips on a serving platter or plate.

3. Serve the tahini dip alongside the bell pepper slices, allowing people to dip the peppers into the dip.

Why this is a great anti-inflammatory option for seniors:

- Bell peppers are rich in vitamin C, an antioxidant that can help reduce inflammation.
- Tahini is made from ground sesame seeds, which are a good source of anti-inflammatory compounds like lignans and sesamin.
- Lemon juice provides additional vitamin C and can help enhance the absorption of the dip's nutrients.
- Garlic and cumin are both spices with potent anti-inflammatory properties.
- The overall combination of vegetables, healthy fats, and anti-inflammatory ingredients makes this a nourishing and beneficial snack for seniors.

This sliced bell pepper and tahini dip is a simple, yet flavorful and nutrient-dense option that can help support healthy inflammation levels in seniors. The crunchy peppers paired with the creamy, savory dip create a satisfying and anti-inflammatory snack.

Feel free to adjust the spices or add additional toppings to suit your taste preferences. Enjoy this refreshing and anti-inflammatory vegetable and dip combination!

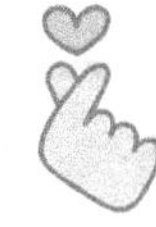

Procedure:

What is the total cooking time, including prep time?

Prep Time : ___________________

Cook Time : ___________________

Servings : ___________________

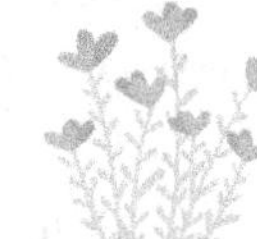

Ingredients:

- 1 bunch of kale, washed and torn into bite-sized pieces (about 4 cups)
- 1 tbsp olive oil
- 2 tbsp nutritional yeast
- 1/2 tsp garlic powder
- 1/4 tsp onion powder
- 1/4 tsp paprika
- Salt and pepper to taste

Is the recipe easy to follow?

20. Kale Chips with Nutritional Yeast

1. Preheat your oven to 325°F (165°C).

2. In a large bowl, toss the kale pieces with the olive oil, making sure to evenly coat the leaves.

3. In a small bowl, mix together the nutritional yeast, garlic powder, onion powder, and paprika.

4. Sprinkle the seasoning mixture over the kale and toss again to distribute the seasoning evenly.

5. Spread the seasoned kale in a single layer on a baking sheet lined with parchment paper.

6. Bake the kale chips in the preheated oven for 12-15 minutes, or until they are crispy and lightly browned.

7. Remove the kale chips from the oven and season with salt and pepper to taste.

8. Allow the kale chips to cool slightly before serving.

Why this is a great anti-inflammatory option for seniors:

- Kale is a nutrient-dense leafy green that is rich in antioxidants and anti-inflammatory compounds like vitamin C, vitamin K, and carotenoids.
- Nutritional yeast is a good source of B vitamins, which can help reduce inflammation.
- Garlic and onion powders have natural anti-inflammatory properties.
- Paprika contains capsaicin, a compound with potent anti-inflammatory effects.

Feel free to adjust the seasoning blend to your personal taste preferences. Enjoy these delicious and anti-inflammatory kale chips!

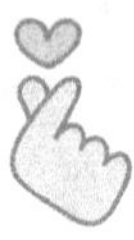

What are the critical points in the recipe (e.g., temperature control, timing)?

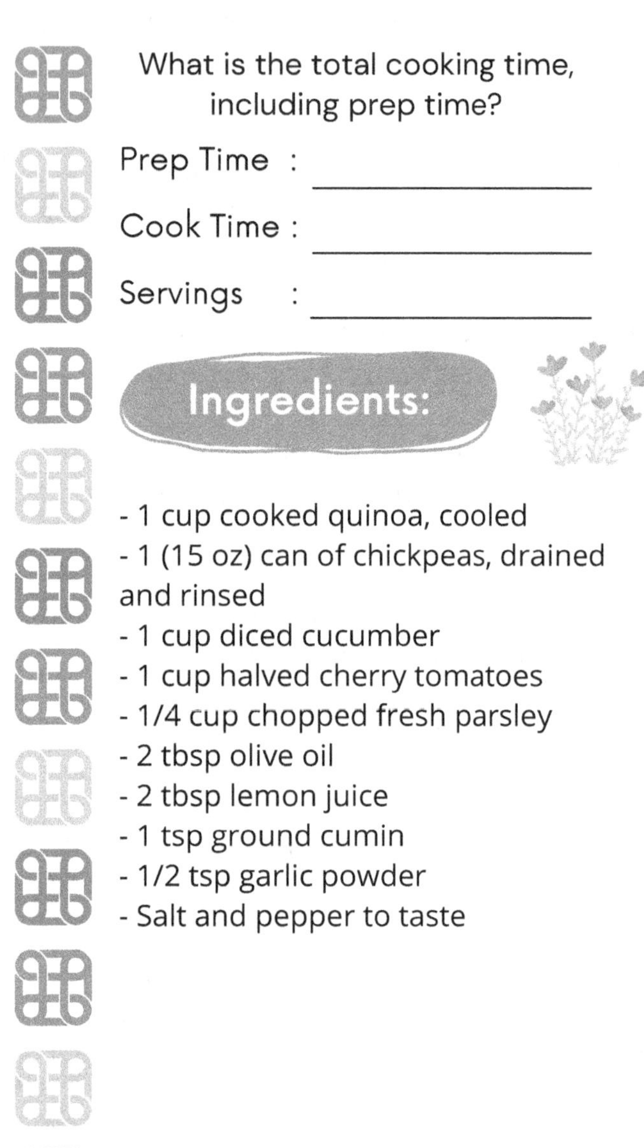

What is the total cooking time, including prep time?

Prep Time : _______________

Cook Time : _______________

Servings   : _______________

Ingredients:

- 1 cup cooked quinoa, cooled
- 1 (15 oz) can of chickpeas, drained and rinsed
- 1 cup diced cucumber
- 1 cup halved cherry tomatoes
- 1/4 cup chopped fresh parsley
- 2 tbsp olive oil
- 2 tbsp lemon juice
- 1 tsp ground cumin
- 1/2 tsp garlic powder
- Salt and pepper to taste

Is the recipe easy to follow?

21. Quinoa Salad with Chickpeas, Cucumbers, and Tomatoes

1. In a large bowl, combine the cooked and cooled quinoa, chickpeas, diced cucumber, halved cherry tomatoes, and chopped parsley.

2. In a small bowl, whisk together the olive oil, lemon juice, cumin, and garlic powder.

3. Pour the dressing over the quinoa salad and toss gently to coat the ingredients evenly.

4. Season the salad with salt and pepper to taste.

5. Refrigerate the quinoa salad for at least 30 minutes to allow the flavors to meld.

6. Serve chilled or at room temperature.

Why this is a great anti-inflammatory option for seniors:

- Quinoa is a whole grain that is high in fiber, protein, and anti-inflammatory nutrients like magnesium and B vitamins.
- Chickpeas are a good source of plant-based protein and contain anti-inflammatory compounds like folate and magnesium.
- Cucumbers are hydrating and contain anti-inflammatory lignans and flavonoids.
- Tomatoes are rich in the antioxidant lycopene, which has potent anti-inflammatory properties.
- Parsley, olive oil, lemon juice, cumin, and garlic are all ingredients with natural anti-inflammatory benefits.

This quinoa salad provides a nutrient-dense, flavorful, and anti-inflammatory meal or snack that can be especially beneficial for seniors. The combination of whole grains, vegetables, and anti-inflammatory ingredients makes it a great choice for supporting overall health and reducing inflammation.

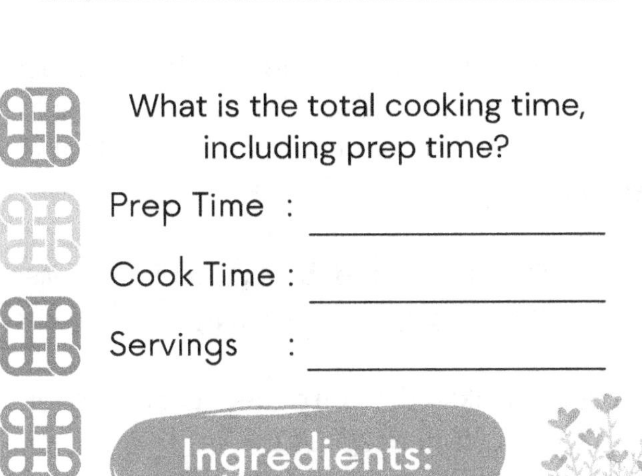

What is the total cooking time, including prep time?

Prep Time : ______________

Cook Time : ______________

Servings   : ______________

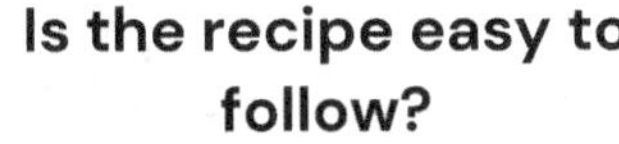

Ingredients:

- 1 cup dry brown or green lentils, rinsed
- 4 cups low-sodium vegetable or chicken broth
- 1 tbsp olive oil
- 1 onion, diced
- 3 garlic cloves, minced
- 1 tbsp ground turmeric
- 1 tsp ground cumin
- 1/2 tsp ground coriander
- 4 cups fresh spinach, chopped
- Salt and pepper to taste
- Lemon wedges for serving (optional)

Is the recipe easy to follow?

22. Lentil Soup with Turmeric and Spinach

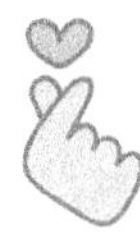

Procedure:

1. In a large pot, combine the rinsed lentils and broth. Bring the mixture to a boil over high heat.

2. Reduce the heat to medium-low, cover, and simmer for 15-20 minutes, or until the lentils are tender.

3. In a separate skillet, heat the olive oil over medium heat. Add the diced onion and sauté for 5-7 minutes, until translucent.

4. Add the minced garlic, turmeric, cumin, and coriander to the skillet. Cook for 1-2 minutes, stirring constantly, until fragrant.

5. Transfer the sautéed onion and spice mixture to the pot with the cooked lentils. Stir to combine.

6. Add the chopped spinach to the pot and stir until the spinach is wilted, about 2-3 minutes.

7. Season the lentil soup with salt and pepper to taste.

8. Serve the lentil soup warm, with a squeeze of lemon juice over the top, if desired.

This lentil soup provides a nourishing, comforting, and anti-inflammatory meal that can be especially beneficial for seniors. The combination of protein-rich lentils, anti-inflammatory spices, and nutrient-dense greens makes it a great choice for supporting healthy inflammation levels.

Feel free to adjust the spices or add other anti-inflammatory vegetables to customize the soup to your liking. Enjoy this delicious and anti-inflammatory lentil soup!

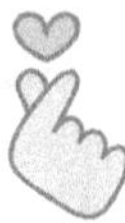

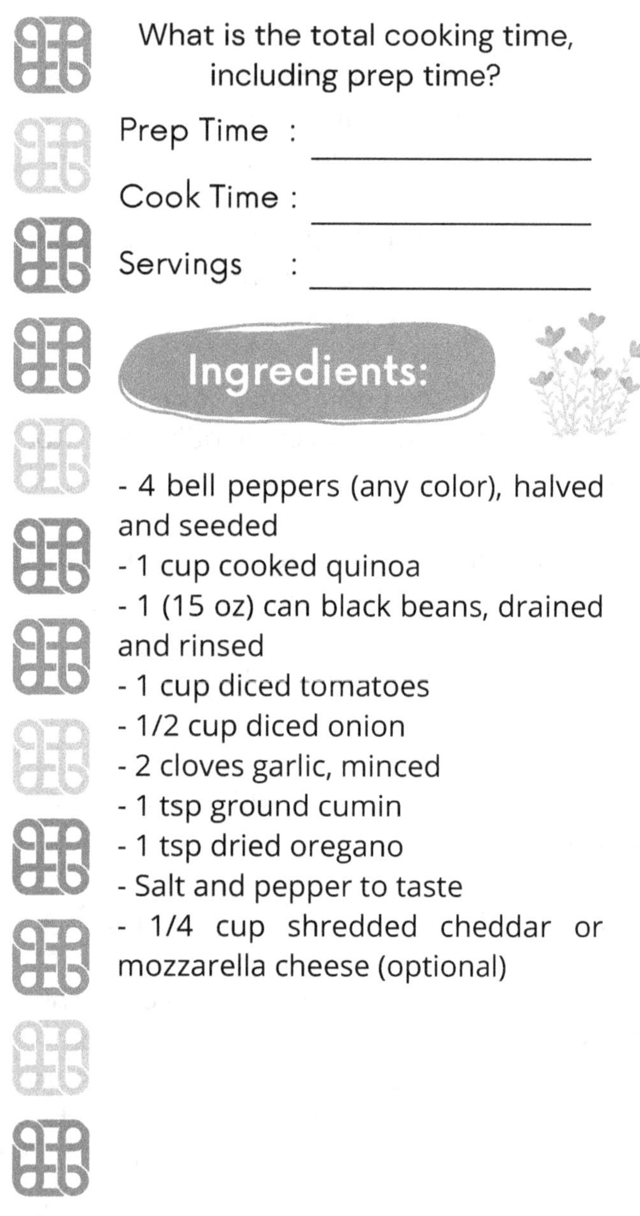

What is the total cooking time, including prep time?

Prep Time : _______________

Cook Time : _______________

Servings : _______________

Ingredients:

- 4 bell peppers (any color), halved and seeded
- 1 cup cooked quinoa
- 1 (15 oz) can black beans, drained and rinsed
- 1 cup diced tomatoes
- 1/2 cup diced onion
- 2 cloves garlic, minced
- 1 tsp ground cumin
- 1 tsp dried oregano
- Salt and pepper to taste
- 1/4 cup shredded cheddar or mozzarella cheese (optional)

Is the recipe easy to follow?

23. Stuffed Bell Peppers with Quinoa and Black Beans

1. Preheat your oven to 375°F (190°C).

2. Arrange the bell pepper halves in a baking dish or on a rimmed baking sheet.

3. In a medium bowl, combine the cooked quinoa, black beans, diced tomatoes, onion, garlic, cumin, and oregano. Season with salt and pepper to taste.

4. Spoon the quinoa and black bean mixture evenly into the bell pepper halves.

5. If using, sprinkle the shredded cheese over the top of the stuffed peppers.

6. Bake the stuffed peppers in the preheated oven for 25-30 minutes, or until the peppers are tender and the filling is heated through.

7. Serve the stuffed bell peppers warm.

Why this is a great anti-inflammatory option for seniors:

- Bell peppers are rich in vitamin C, an antioxidant with anti-inflammatory properties.
- Quinoa is a whole grain that is high in fiber, protein, and anti-inflammatory nutrients like magnesium and B vitamins.
- Black beans are a good source of plant-based protein and contain anti-inflammatory compounds like anthocyanins.
- Tomatoes are rich in the antioxidant lycopene, which has potent anti-inflammatory effects.
- Onions and garlic are both natural anti-inflammatory ingredients.
- Cumin and oregano are spices with their own anti-inflammatory benefits.

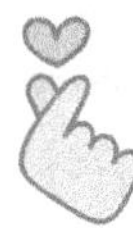

What are the critical points in the recipe (e.g., temperature control, timing)?

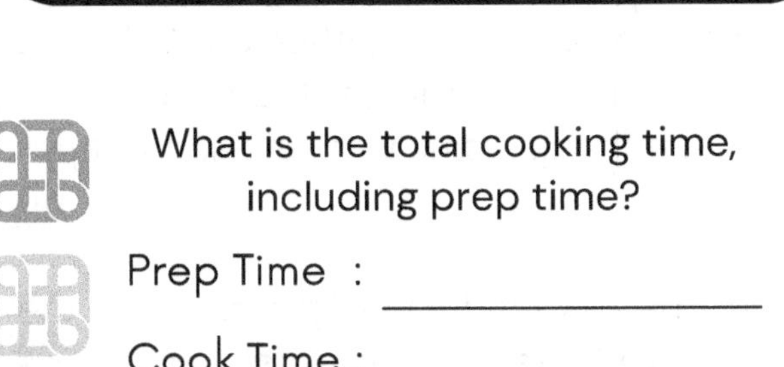

What is the total cooking time, including prep time?

Prep Time : _________________

Cook Time : _________________

Servings   : _________________

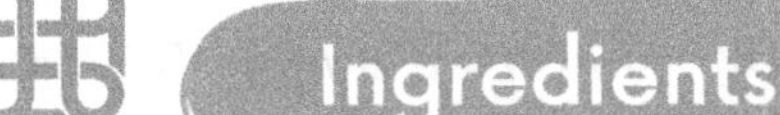

Ingredients:

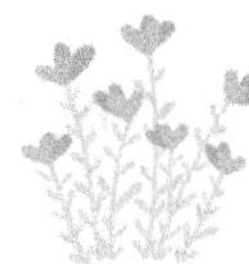

For the Buddha Bowl:
- 1 medium sweet potato, peeled and cubed
- 1 cup cooked quinoa
- 1 cup cooked chickpeas
- 1 cup baby spinach
- 1/2 cup diced cucumber
- 2 tbsp toasted pumpkin seeds

For the Tahini Dressing:
- 2 tbsp tahini
- 2 tbsp freshly squeezed lemon juice
- 1 tbsp water
- 1 tsp ground cumin
- 1 garlic clove, minced
- Salt and pepper to taste

Is the recipe easy to follow?

24. Vegan Buddha Bowl with Sweet Potatoes and Tahini Dressing

1. Preheat your oven to 400°F (200°C). Toss the cubed sweet potato with a drizzle of olive oil and roast for 20-25 minutes, or until tender.

2. In a large bowl, combine the roasted sweet potato, cooked quinoa, chickpeas, baby spinach, and diced cucumber.

3. In a small bowl, whisk together the tahini, lemon juice, water, cumin, and minced garlic. Season the tahini dressing with salt and pepper to taste.

4. Drizzle the tahini dressing over the Buddha bowl and sprinkle the toasted pumpkin seeds on top. Serve the Vegan Buddha Bowl immediately.

Why this is a great anti-inflammatory option for seniors:

- Sweet potatoes are rich in anti-inflammatory beta-carotene and vitamin C.
- Quinoa is a whole grain that provides anti-inflammatory nutrients like magnesium and B vitamins.
- Chickpeas are a good source of plant-based protein and contain anti-inflammatory compounds like folate.
- Spinach is packed with antioxidants and anti-inflammatory vitamins like vitamin K and vitamin C.
- Tahini is made from ground sesame seeds, which are a source of anti-inflammatory lignans.
- Lemon juice, cumin, and garlic all have natural anti-inflammatory properties.
- Pumpkin seeds are rich in anti-inflammatory omega-3 fatty acids.

What are the critical points in the recipe (e.g., temperature control, timing)?

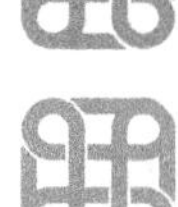 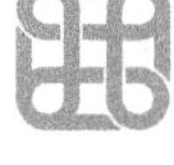 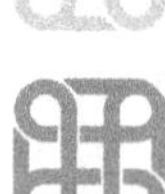 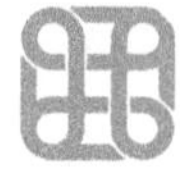

What is the total cooking time, including prep time?

Prep Time : _______________

Cook Time : _______________

Servings   : _______________

Ingredients:

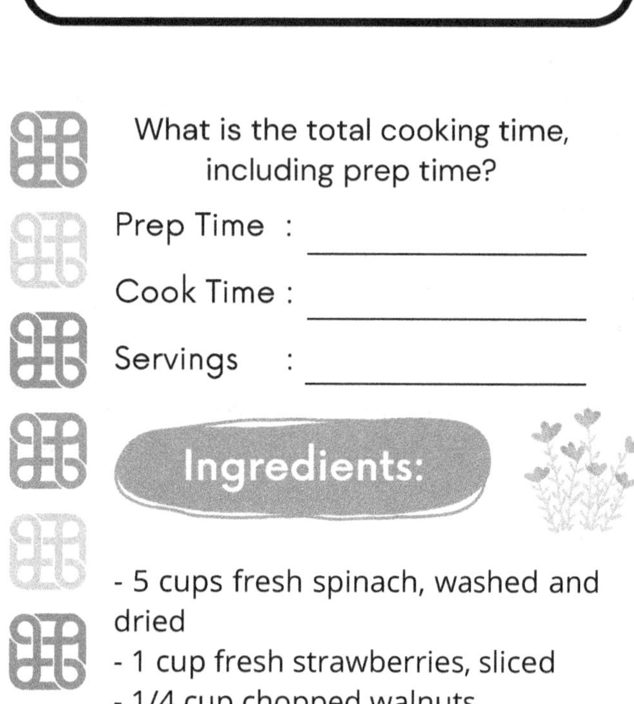

- 5 cups fresh spinach, washed and dried
- 1 cup fresh strawberries, sliced
- 1/4 cup chopped walnuts
- 2 tbsp balsamic vinegar
- 1 tbsp extra-virgin olive oil
- 1 tsp Dijon mustard
- 1 tsp honey (optional)
- Salt and pepper to taste

Is the recipe easy to follow?

25. Spinach and Strawberry Salad with Walnuts

Procedure:

1. In a large salad bowl, combine the fresh spinach, sliced strawberries, and chopped walnuts.

2. In a small bowl, whisk together the balsamic vinegar, olive oil, Dijon mustard, and honey (if using). Season the dressing with salt and pepper to taste.

3. Drizzle the balsamic vinaigrette over the spinach, strawberries, and walnuts. Gently toss to coat the salad ingredients evenly. Serve the Spinach and Strawberry Salad immediately.

Why this is a great anti-inflammatory option for seniors:

- Spinach is a nutrient-dense leafy green that is rich in antioxidants and anti-inflammatory compounds like vitamin C, vitamin K, and carotenoids.
- Strawberries are packed with anti-inflammatory anthocyanins and vitamin C.
- Walnuts are a good source of anti-inflammatory omega-3 fatty acids, as well as antioxidants.
- Balsamic vinegar contains polyphenols that can help reduce inflammation.
- Olive oil is a healthy fat with anti-inflammatory properties.
- Dijon mustard and honey (if used) can also provide some anti-inflammatory benefits.

This Spinach and Strawberry Salad with Walnuts is a refreshing, flavorful, and nutrient-dense option that can be especially beneficial for seniors. The combination of antioxidant-rich greens, anti-inflammatory berries, and healthy fats from the walnuts and olive oil makes it a great choice for supporting healthy inflammation levels.

Procedure:

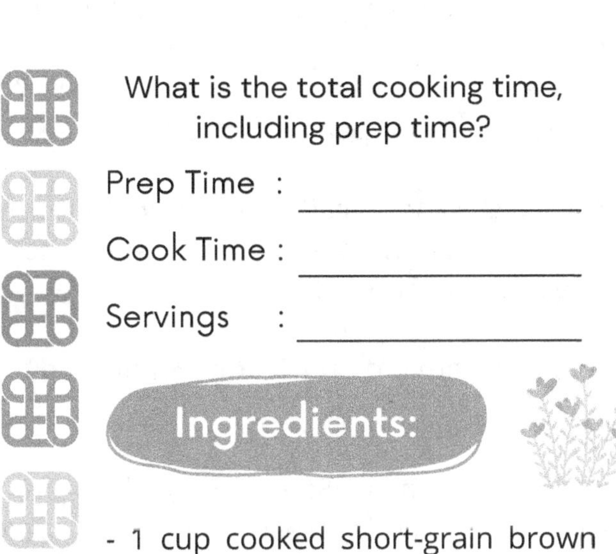

What is the total cooking time, including prep time?

Prep Time : ________________

Cook Time : ________________

Servings : ________________

Ingredients:

- 1 cup cooked short-grain brown rice
- 2 tbsp rice vinegar
- 1 tsp sugar
- 1/4 tsp salt
- 1 avocado, sliced
- 1 cucumber, peeled and cut into thin strips
- 4-6 sheets of nori (seaweed sheets)
- Wasabi and low-sodium soy sauce, for serving (optional)

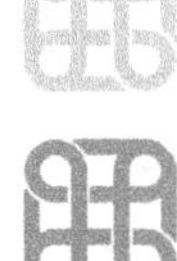
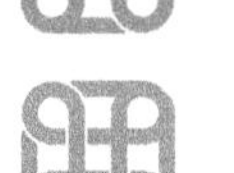

Is the recipe easy to follow?

26. Vegan Sushi Rolls with Avocado and Cucumber

1. In a medium bowl, combine the cooked brown rice, rice vinegar, sugar, and salt. Stir until the sugar and salt have dissolved.

2. Lay a sheet of nori on a bamboo sushi mat or clean, flat surface. Spread about 1/4 cup of the seasoned rice evenly over the nori, leaving a 1-inch border at the top.

3. Arrange a few slices of avocado and cucumber strips in a line across the center of the rice.

4. Carefully roll the nori around the fillings, using the bamboo mat to help you roll it tightly. Moisten the top edge of the nori with a bit of water to seal the roll.

5. Repeat the process with the remaining nori sheets and fillings.

6. Using a sharp knife, slice each sushi roll into 6-8 pieces. Serve the vegan sushi rolls with wasabi and low-sodium soy sauce, if desired.

Why this is a great anti-inflammatory option for seniors:

- Avocado is rich in healthy monounsaturated fats, which have anti-inflammatory properties.
- Cucumber is hydrating and contains anti-inflammatory compounds like lignans and flavonoids.
- Brown rice is a whole grain that provides anti-inflammatory nutrients like magnesium and B vitamins.
- Nori (seaweed) is a good source of iodine, which can help regulate inflammation.
- The overall combination of healthy fats, vegetables, and whole grains makes this a nutrient-dense and anti-inflammatory meal option.

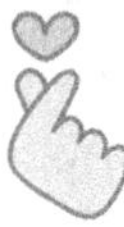

What is the total cooking time, including prep time?

Prep Time : _______________

Cook Time : _______________

Servings   : _______________

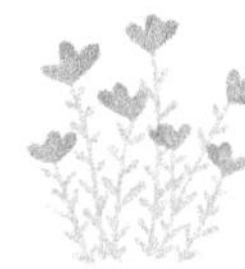

Ingredients:

- 1 (15 oz) can chickpeas, drained and rinsed
- 2 tablespoons mayonnaise
- 1 tablespoon Dijon mustard
- 1 tablespoon lemon juice
- 1/4 cup diced celery
- 2 tablespoons diced red onion
- 1 tablespoon chopped fresh parsley
- Salt and pepper to taste
- 4 slices whole grain bread

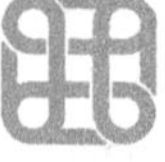
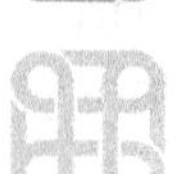
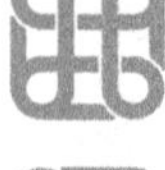
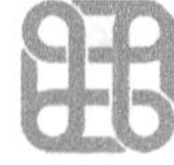

Is the recipe easy to follow?

27. Chickpea Salad Sandwich on Whole Grain Bread

1. In a medium bowl, mash the chickpeas with a fork or potato masher until slightly chunky.

2. Add the mayonnaise, Dijon mustard, lemon juice, celery, red onion, and parsley. Stir to combine.

3. Season with salt and pepper to taste.

4. Spread the chickpea salad evenly onto 2 slices of the whole grain bread. Top with the remaining 2 slices of bread.

5. Serve immediately or refrigerate until ready to eat.

Enjoy your Chickpea Salad Sandwich on wholesome whole grain bread! The chickpeas provide protein, fiber, and nutrients, while the whole grains offer complex carbohydrates for sustained energy.

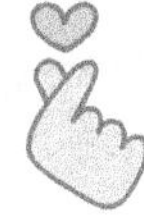

What is the total cooking time, including prep time?

Prep Time : _________________

Cook Time : _________________

Servings : _________________

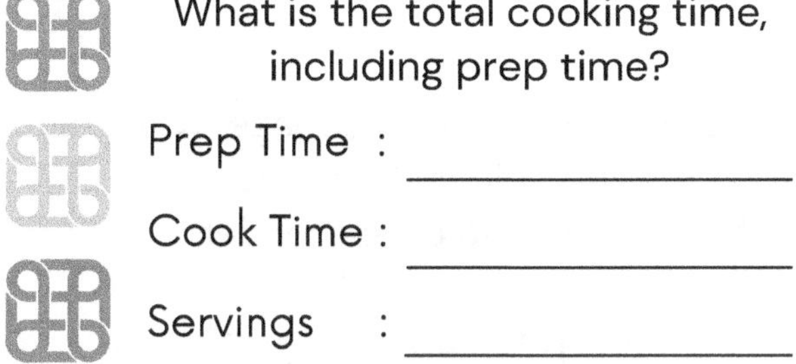

Ingredients:

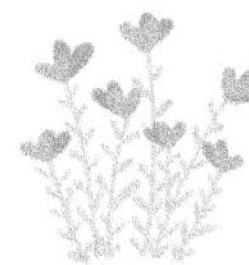

- 1 cup uncooked quinoa, rinsed
- 2 cups low-sodium vegetable broth
- 1 medium sweet potato, peeled and diced
- 1 red bell pepper, diced
- 1 zucchini, diced
- 1 red onion, diced
- 2 tablespoons olive oil
- 1 teaspoon ground cumin
- 1/2 teaspoon garlic powder
- Salt and pepper to taste
- 2 cups baby spinach
- 1/4 cup chopped fresh parsley
- 2 tablespoons toasted pumpkin seeds
- 2 tablespoons balsamic vinegar

Is the recipe easy to follow?

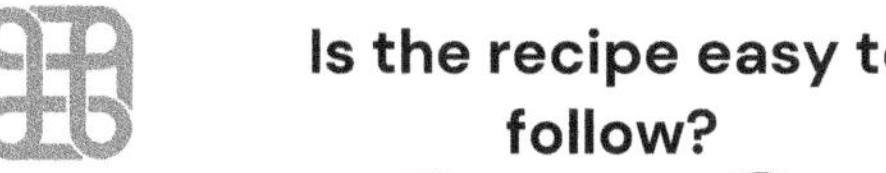

28. Roasted Vegetable and Quinoa Salad

1. Preheat oven to 400°F. Toss the sweet potato, bell pepper, zucchini, and onion with the olive oil, cumin, garlic powder, salt and pepper. Spread on a baking sheet and roast for 20-25 minutes, until tender.

2. Meanwhile, cook the quinoa according to package directions using the vegetable broth. Fluff with a fork and let cool slightly.

3. In a large bowl, combine the roasted vegetables, cooked quinoa, spinach, parsley, and pumpkin seeds.

4. Drizzle the balsamic vinegar over the salad and toss gently to coat.

5. Serve immediately or refrigerate until ready to serve.

This salad is packed with anti-inflammatory ingredients like quinoa, vegetables, and healthy fats from the olive oil and pumpkin seeds. The fiber, protein, and complex carbs make it a nutritious and filling meal for seniors. Adjust seasoning to taste.

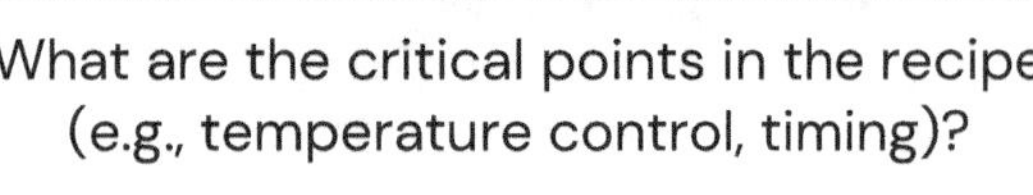

What are the critical points in the recipe (e.g., temperature control, timing)?

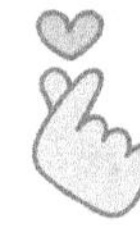

1. In a medium saucepan, bring the broth to a simmer over medium heat.

2. In a small bowl, whisk a few tablespoons of the hot broth into the miso paste until smooth. Then whisk the miso mixture back into the saucepan.

3. Add the tofu, mushrooms, cabbage, wakame, green onions, and ginger. Simmer for 5-7 minutes, until the vegetables are tender.

4. Season with salt and pepper to taste.

5. Ladle the soup into bowls and serve hot.

This miso soup is packed with anti-inflammatory ingredients like tofu, mushrooms, cabbage, and wakame seaweed. The miso paste provides probiotics, while the ginger adds anti-inflammatory properties. It's a nourishing, low-calorie soup that's easy to digest for seniors. Adjust seasoning and ingredients to your taste preferences.

What is the total cooking time, including prep time?

Prep Time : ________________

Cook Time : ________________

Servings   : ________________

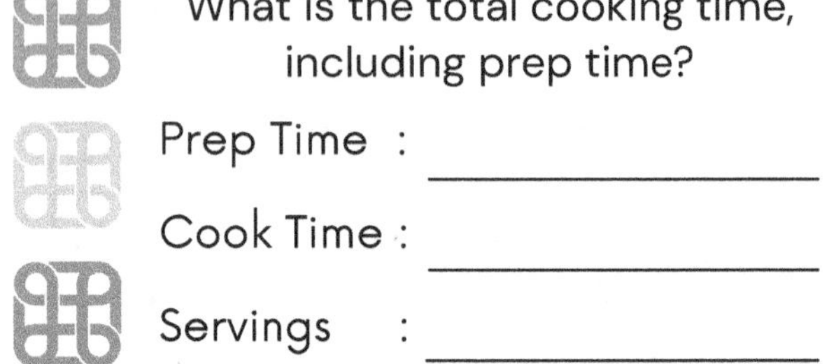

- 4 cups low-sodium vegetable or chicken broth
- 2 tablespoons white or yellow miso paste
- 1 (12 oz) block firm or extra-firm tofu, cubed
- 1 cup thinly sliced shiitake mushrooms
- 1 cup thinly sliced napa cabbage
- 2 tablespoons dried wakame seaweed
- 2 green onions, thinly sliced
- 1 teaspoon grated fresh ginger
- Salt and pepper to taste

Is the recipe easy to follow?

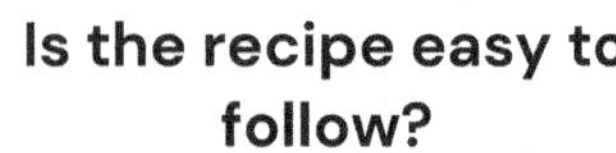

29. Miso Soup with Tofu and Seaweed

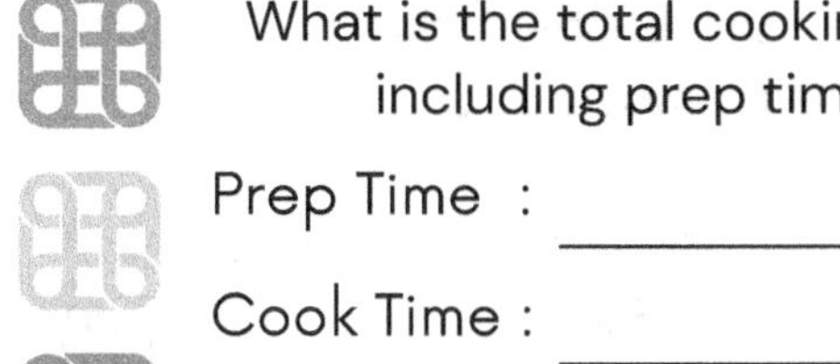

What is the total cooking time, including prep time?

Prep Time : _______________

Cook Time : _______________

Servings   : _______________

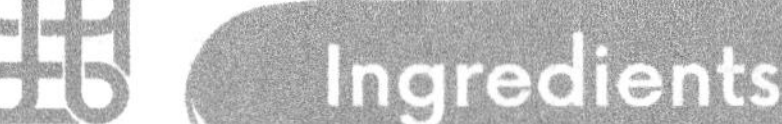
Ingredients:

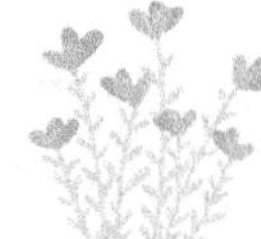

- 1 head of cauliflower, riced (about 4 cups riced cauliflower)
- 1 tablespoon sesame oil
- 1 block (14 oz) extra-firm tofu, cubed
- 2 cloves garlic, minced
- 1 tablespoon grated fresh ginger
- 1 red bell pepper, thinly sliced
- 1 cup sliced mushrooms
- 2 cups baby spinach
- 2 tablespoons low-sodium soy sauce or tamari
- 1 tablespoon rice vinegar
- 1 teaspoon sesame seeds
- Salt and pepper to taste

Is the recipe easy to follow?

30. Cauliflower Rice Stir-Fry with Tofu

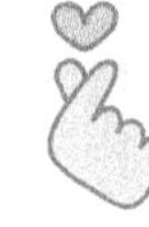

Procedure:

1. If using a whole head of cauliflower, pulse it in a food processor until it resembles rice-sized grains. Measure out 4 cups of riced cauliflower.

2. Heat the sesame oil in a large skillet or wok over medium-high heat. Add the tofu cubes and cook for 3-4 minutes per side until lightly browned. Transfer the tofu to a plate.

3. Add the garlic and ginger to the skillet and cook for 1 minute, until fragrant.

4. Add the riced cauliflower, bell pepper, and mushrooms. Stir-fry for 5-7 minutes, until the vegetables are tender-crisp.

5. Stir in the spinach, soy sauce, and rice vinegar. Cook for 1-2 minutes until the spinach is wilted.

6. Return the tofu to the skillet and toss everything together.

7. Sprinkle with sesame seeds and season with salt and pepper to taste.

8. Serve hot.

This cauliflower rice stir-fry is packed with anti-inflammatory ingredients like cauliflower, bell pepper, mushrooms, spinach, ginger, and tofu. The healthy fats from the sesame oil and sesame seeds also provide anti-inflammatory benefits. It's a nutritious, low-carb meal for seniors.

What are the critical points in the recipe (e.g., temperature control, timing)?

What is the total cooking time, including prep time?

Prep Time : ______________

Cook Time : ______________

Servings : ______________

Ingredients:

- 4 medium sweet potatoes
- 1 (15 oz) can black beans, drained and rinsed
- 1 avocado, diced
- 2 tablespoons olive oil
- 1 teaspoon ground cumin
- 1 teaspoon chili powder
- 1/4 cup chopped fresh cilantro
- Juice of 1 lime
- Salt and pepper to taste

Is the recipe easy to follow?

31. Baked Sweet Potato with Black Beans and Avocado

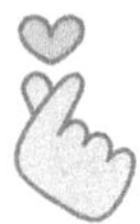

Procedure:

1. Preheat the oven to 400°F. Pierce the sweet potatoes several times with a fork and place them directly on the oven rack. Bake for 45-60 minutes, until very soft when squeezed.

2. In a medium bowl, combine the black beans, avocado, olive oil, cumin, chili powder, cilantro, and lime juice. Season with salt and pepper.

3. Once the sweet potatoes are cooked, let them cool for 5 minutes. Slice each one open lengthwise.

4. Scoop out about 2-3 tablespoons of the sweet potato flesh from the center of each potato, leaving a thin layer attached to the skin.

5. Mash the scooped-out sweet potato flesh and fold it into the black bean and avocado mixture.

6. Spoon the black bean and avocado mixture back into the sweet potato skins.

7. Serve the stuffed sweet potatoes warm.

This dish is packed with anti-inflammatory ingredients like sweet potatoes, black beans, avocado, and spices. The healthy fats, fiber, and complex carbs make it a nutritious and satisfying meal for seniors. Adjust seasoning to your taste preferences.

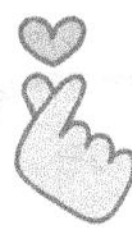

Procedure:

What is the total cooking time, including prep time?

Prep Time : _________________

Cook Time : _________________

Servings : _________________

Ingredients:

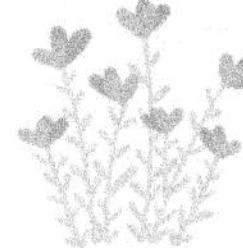

- 1 cup uncooked brown rice
- 1 tablespoon olive oil
- 1 onion, diced
- 3 cloves garlic, minced
- 1 tablespoon grated fresh ginger
- 1 teaspoon ground cumin
- 1 teaspoon ground coriander
- 1 teaspoon turmeric
- 1/2 teaspoon ground cinnamon
- 1/4 teaspoon cayenne pepper (optional)
- 1 (15 oz) can chickpeas, drained and rinsed
- 1 (14 oz) can diced tomatoes
- 1 cup low-sodium vegetable broth
- 4 cups fresh spinach
- 1/4 cup chopped fresh cilantro
- Salt and pepper to taste

Is the recipe easy to follow?

32. Chickpea and Spinach Curry with Brown Rice

1. Cook the brown rice according to package directions.

2. In a large skillet or pot, heat the olive oil over medium heat. Add the onion and sauté for 5 minutes until translucent.

3. Add the garlic, ginger, cumin, coriander, turmeric, cinnamon, and cayenne (if using). Cook for 1 minute until fragrant.

4. Stir in the chickpeas, diced tomatoes, and vegetable broth. Bring to a simmer and cook for 10 minutes.

5. Add the spinach and cook for 2-3 minutes until wilted.

6. Remove from heat and stir in the chopped cilantro. Season with salt and pepper to taste.

7. Serve the chickpea curry over the cooked brown rice.

This curry is packed with anti-inflammatory ingredients like chickpeas, spinach, ginger, and turmeric. The complex carbs from the brown rice provide sustained energy. It's a nourishing, flavorful meal for seniors. Adjust spice level to your preference.

What are the critical points in the recipe (e.g., temperature control, timing)?

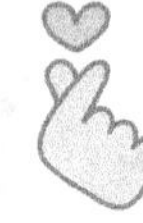

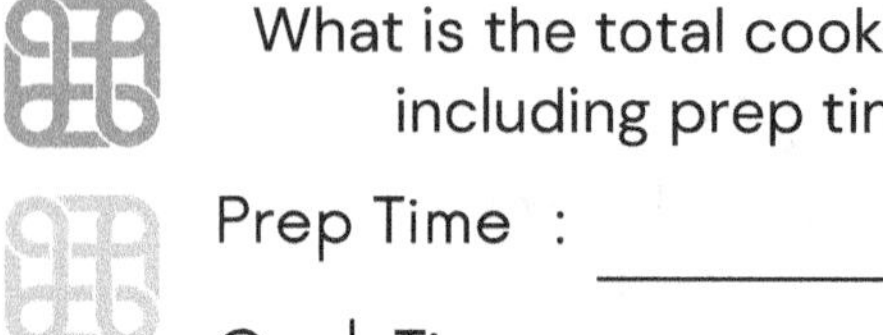

What is the total cooking time, including prep time?

Prep Time : ______________

Cook Time : ______________

Servings   : ______________

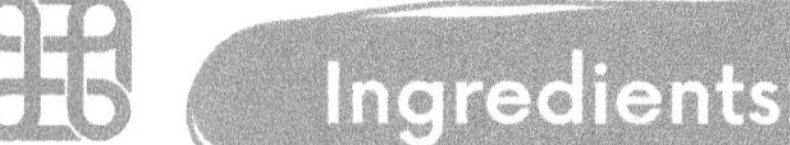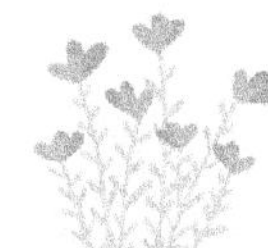

Ingredients:

- 2 acorn squash, halved and seeded
- 1 cup uncooked quinoa, rinsed
- 2 cups low-sodium vegetable broth
- 1/2 cup dried cranberries
- 1/4 cup chopped walnuts
- 2 tablespoons olive oil
- 1 teaspoon ground cinnamon
- 1/2 teaspoon ground ginger
- 1/4 teaspoon ground nutmeg
- Salt and pepper to taste
- 2 tablespoons chopped fresh parsley

Is the recipe easy to follow?

33. Stuffed Acorn Squash with Quinoa and Cranberries

1. Preheat the oven to 400°F. Place the acorn squash halves cut-side up on a baking sheet. Roast for 30-40 minutes, until tender when pierced with a fork.

2. Meanwhile, in a medium saucepan, combine the quinoa and vegetable broth. Bring to a boil, then reduce heat, cover and simmer for 15-20 minutes until quinoa is cooked through. Fluff with a fork.

3. In a medium bowl, mix the cooked quinoa, cranberries, walnuts, olive oil, cinnamon, ginger, nutmeg, and salt and pepper to taste.

4. Once the squash is tender, scoop the quinoa mixture into the squash halves, dividing it evenly.

5. Return the stuffed squash to the oven and bake for an additional 10-15 minutes, until heated through.

6. Garnish with chopped fresh parsley before serving.

This stuffed squash dish is packed with anti-inflammatory ingredients like acorn squash, quinoa, cranberries, walnuts, and warming spices. The fiber, complex carbs, and healthy fats make it a nutritious and satisfying meal for seniors. Adjust seasoning to your taste preferences.

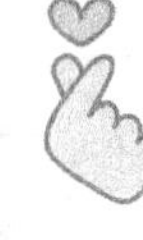

Procedure:

What is the total cooking time, including prep time?

Prep Time : _______________

Cook Time : _______________

Servings   : _______________

Ingredients:

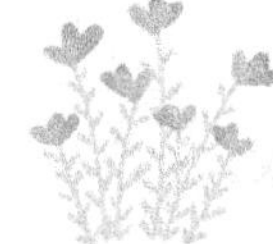

- 1 tablespoon olive oil
- 1 onion, diced
- 3 cloves garlic, minced
- 2 carrots, peeled and diced
- 2 stalks celery, diced
- 1 cup brown or green lentils, rinsed
- 4 cups low-sodium vegetable or chicken broth
- 1 (14 oz) can diced tomatoes
- 1 bay leaf
- 1 teaspoon dried thyme
- 1/2 teaspoon ground cumin
- Salt and pepper to taste
- 2 cups baby spinach
- 2 tablespoons chopped fresh parsley

Is the recipe easy to follow?

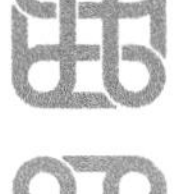

34. Lentil Stew with Carrots and Celery

1. In a large pot or Dutch oven, heat the olive oil over medium heat. Add the onion and sauté for 5 minutes until translucent.

2. Add the garlic, carrots, and celery. Cook for 3-4 minutes, stirring frequently, until the vegetables start to soften.

3. Stir in the lentils, broth, diced tomatoes, bay leaf, thyme, and cumin. Season with salt and pepper.

4. Bring the stew to a boil, then reduce heat and simmer for 25-30 minutes, until the lentils are tender.

5. Remove the bay leaf. Stir in the baby spinach and let it wilt for 2-3 minutes.

6. Ladle the lentil stew into bowls and garnish with chopped fresh parsley.

This lentil stew is packed with anti-inflammatory ingredients like lentils, carrots, celery, spinach, and herbs. The fiber, protein, and complex carbs make it a nourishing and filling meal for seniors. Adjust seasoning to your taste preferences.

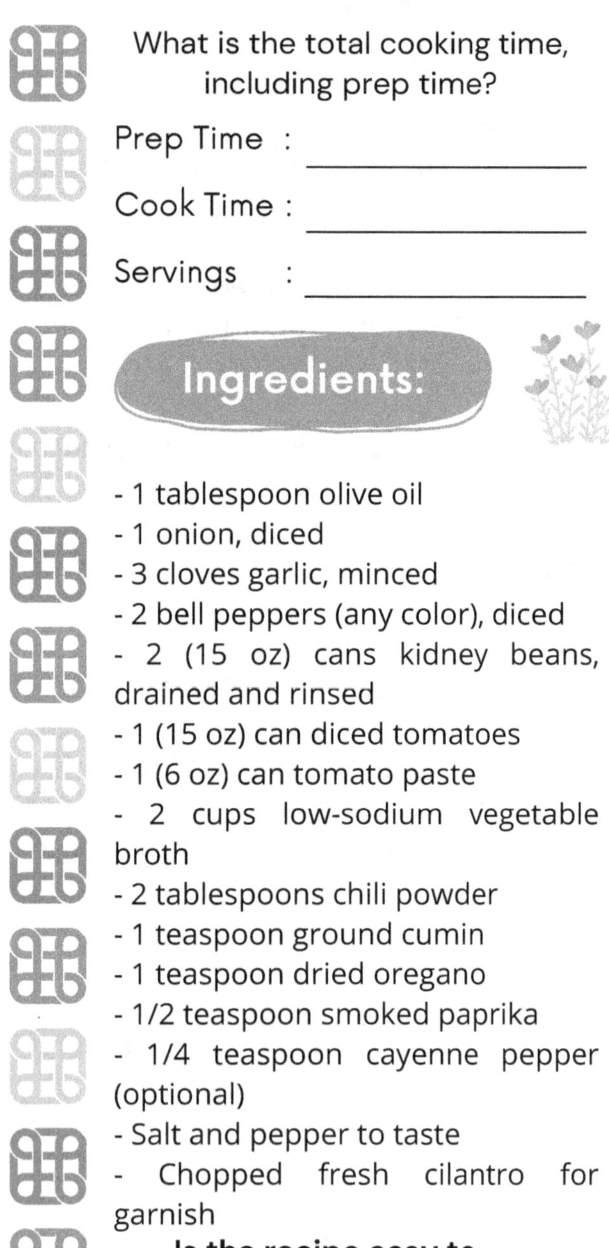

What is the total cooking time, including prep time?

Prep Time : _______________

Cook Time : _______________

Servings   : _______________

Ingredients:

- 1 tablespoon olive oil
- 1 onion, diced
- 3 cloves garlic, minced
- 2 bell peppers (any color), diced
- 2 (15 oz) cans kidney beans, drained and rinsed
- 1 (15 oz) can diced tomatoes
- 1 (6 oz) can tomato paste
- 2 cups low-sodium vegetable broth
- 2 tablespoons chili powder
- 1 teaspoon ground cumin
- 1 teaspoon dried oregano
- 1/2 teaspoon smoked paprika
- 1/4 teaspoon cayenne pepper (optional)
- Salt and pepper to taste
- Chopped fresh cilantro for garnish

Is the recipe easy to follow?

☺   ☹

35. Vegan Chili with Kidney Beans and Bell Peppers

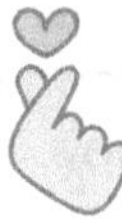

Procedure:

1. In a large pot or Dutch oven, heat the olive oil over medium heat. Add the onion and sauté for 5 minutes until translucent.

2. Add the garlic and bell peppers. Cook for 3-4 minutes, stirring frequently, until the peppers start to soften.

3. Stir in the kidney beans, diced tomatoes, tomato paste, vegetable broth, chili powder, cumin, oregano, smoked paprika, and cayenne (if using). Season with salt and pepper.

4. Bring the chili to a simmer and let it cook for 20-25 minutes, stirring occasionally, until thickened.

5. Taste and adjust seasonings as needed.

6. Ladle the chili into bowls and garnish with chopped fresh cilantro.

This vegan chili is packed with anti-inflammatory ingredients like kidney beans, bell peppers, tomatoes, and spices. The fiber, protein, and complex carbs make it a hearty and nutritious meal for seniors. Adjust the spice level to your preference.

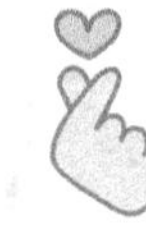

What are the critical points in the recipe (e.g., temperature control, timing)?

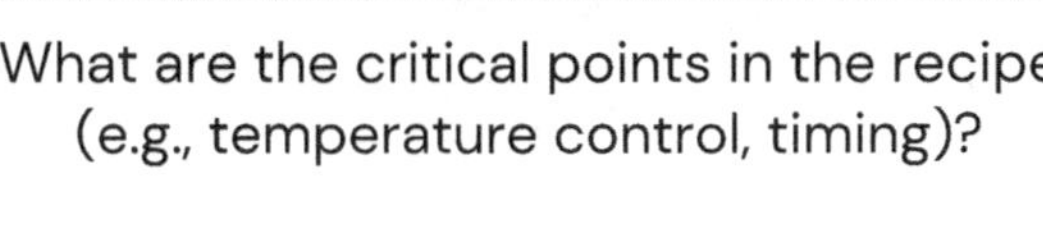 What is the total cooking time, including prep time?

Prep Time : _______________

Cook Time : _______________

Servings : _______________

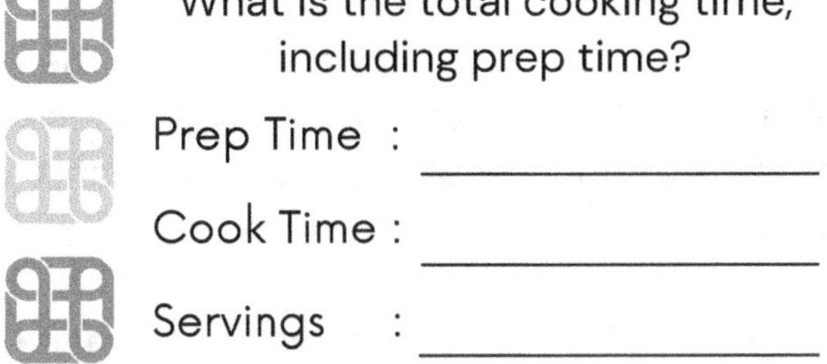

Ingredients:

For the Quinoa Salad:
- 1 cup uncooked quinoa, rinsed
- 2 cups low-sodium vegetable broth
- 1 cup diced cucumber
- 1 cup diced tomatoes
- 1/2 cup diced red onion
- 1/4 cup chopped fresh parsley
- 2 tablespoons olive oil
- 2 tablespoons lemon juice
- 1/2 teaspoon ground cumin
- Salt and pepper to taste

For the Grilled Portobellos:
- 4 large portobello mushroom caps, stems removed
- 2 tablespoons olive oil
- 1 tablespoon balsamic vinegar
- 1 teaspoon dried thyme
- Salt and pepper to taste

Is the recipe easy to follow?

36. Grilled Portobello Mushrooms with Quinoa Salad

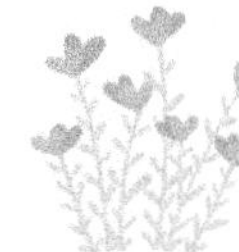

1. Cook the quinoa: In a medium saucepan, combine the quinoa and vegetable broth. Bring to a boil, then reduce heat, cover and simmer for 15-20 minutes until quinoa is cooked through. Fluff with a fork and let cool slightly.

2. Make the quinoa salad: In a large bowl, combine the cooked quinoa, cucumber, tomatoes, red onion, parsley, olive oil, lemon juice, cumin, salt and pepper. Toss to mix well.

3. Prepare the grilled portobellos: Preheat grill or grill pan to medium-high heat. Brush the mushroom caps all over with the olive oil and balsamic vinegar. Sprinkle with the dried thyme, salt and pepper.

4. Grill the mushrooms for 4-5 minutes per side, until tender and lightly charred.

5. Serve the grilled portobello mushrooms warm, topped with the quinoa salad.

This dish is packed with anti-inflammatory ingredients like portobello mushrooms, quinoa, vegetables, and healthy fats from the olive oil. The fiber, protein, and complex carbs make it a nutritious and satisfying meal for seniors. Adjust seasoning to your taste preferences.

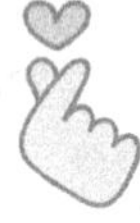

What is the total cooking time, including prep time?

Prep Time : _________________

Cook Time : _________________

Servings   : _________________

Ingredients:

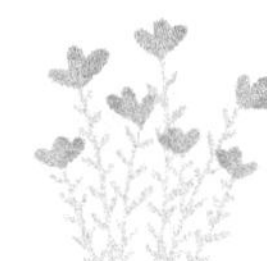

- 2 cups diced sweet potatoes
- 1 red bell pepper, diced
- 1 zucchini, diced
- 1 red onion, diced
- 2 tablespoons olive oil
- 1 teaspoon chili powder
- 1/2 teaspoon ground cumin
- Salt and pepper to taste
- 8-10 small corn tortillas
- 1 avocado, sliced
- 1/4 cup crumbled feta cheese (optional)
- Chopped fresh cilantro for garnish

Is the recipe easy to follow?

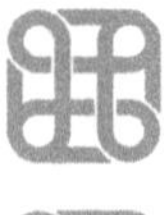

37. Roasted Vegetable Tacos with Avocado

1. Preheat oven to 400°F. Line a baking sheet with parchment paper.

2. In a large bowl, toss the sweet potatoes, bell pepper, zucchini, and onion with the olive oil, chili powder, cumin, salt and pepper.

3. Spread the vegetables in a single layer on the prepared baking sheet. Roast for 20-25 minutes, stirring halfway, until vegetables are tender and lightly browned.

4. Warm the corn tortillas according to package instructions.

5. To assemble the tacos, place some of the roasted vegetables in each tortilla. Top with sliced avocado, crumbled feta (if using), and chopped cilantro.

6. Serve the tacos immediately.

These roasted vegetable tacos are packed with anti-inflammatory ingredients like sweet potatoes, bell peppers, zucchini, and avocado. The healthy fats, fiber, and complex carbs make this a nutritious and satisfying meal for seniors. Adjust the spices and toppings to your taste preferences.

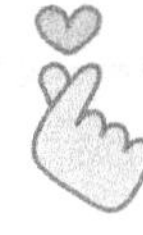

What is the total cooking time, including prep time?

Prep Time : _______________

Cook Time : _______________

Servings : _______________

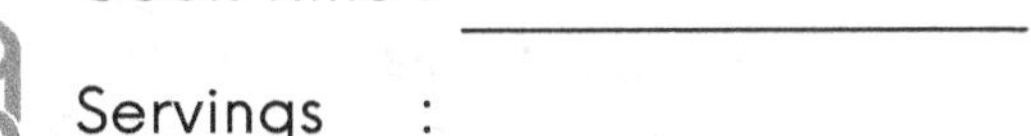

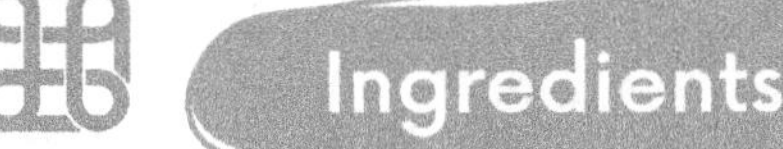
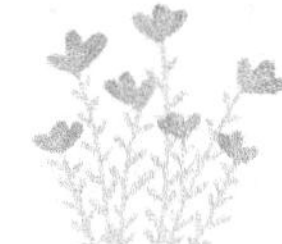

- 1 medium eggplant, diced
- 1 (15 oz) can chickpeas, drained and rinsed
- 1 onion, diced
- 3 cloves garlic, minced
- 1 tablespoon olive oil
- 1 teaspoon ground cumin
- 1 teaspoon smoked paprika
- 1/2 teaspoon ground coriander
- 1 (14 oz) can diced tomatoes
- 1 cup low-sodium vegetable broth
- 2 cups baby spinach
- 2 tablespoons chopped fresh parsley
- Salt and pepper to taste

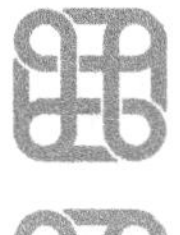

Is the recipe easy to follow?

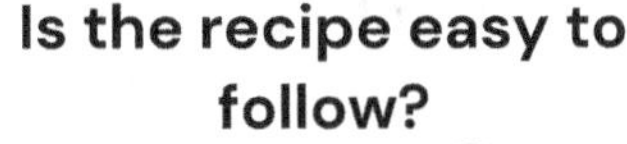

38. Eggplant and Chickpea Stew

1. In a large pot or Dutch oven, heat the olive oil over medium heat. Add the onion and sauté for 5 minutes until translucent.

2. Add the garlic, cumin, smoked paprika, and coriander. Cook for 1 minute, stirring constantly, until fragrant.

3. Stir in the diced eggplant, chickpeas, diced tomatoes, and vegetable broth. Season with salt and pepper.

4. Bring the stew to a simmer and cook for 20-25 minutes, stirring occasionally, until the eggplant is very tender.

5. Stir in the baby spinach and cook for 2-3 minutes until wilted.

6. Remove from heat and stir in the chopped parsley.

7. Serve the eggplant and chickpea stew warm.

This stew is packed with anti-inflammatory ingredients like eggplant, chickpeas, spinach, and aromatic spices. The fiber, protein, and complex carbs make it a nourishing and filling meal for seniors. Adjust seasoning to your taste preferences.

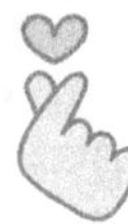

Procedure:

What is the total cooking time, including prep time?

Prep Time : _______________

Cook Time : _______________

Servings : _______________

Ingredients:

For the Filling:
- 1 cup brown or green lentils, rinsed
- 3 cups low-sodium vegetable broth
- 1 onion, diced
- 3 cloves garlic, minced
- 2 carrots, peeled and diced
- 2 stalks celery, diced
- 1 cup frozen peas
- 2 tablespoons tomato paste
- 1 teaspoon dried thyme
- 1 teaspoon dried rosemary
- Salt and pepper to taste

For the Topping:
- 2 lbs Yukon Gold potatoes, peeled and cut into 1-inch chunks
- 1/4 cup unsweetened almond milk
- 2 tablespoons olive oil
- Salt and pepper to taste

39. Vegan Shepherd's Pie with Lentils

1. Preheat oven to 375°F.

2. In a medium saucepan, combine the lentils and vegetable broth. Bring to a boil, then reduce heat and simmer for 20-25 minutes, until lentils are tender. Drain any excess liquid.

3. In a large skillet, sauté the onion and garlic in a bit of olive oil over medium heat for 5 minutes.

4. Add the carrots, celery, peas, tomato paste, thyme, rosemary, salt and pepper. Cook for 10 minutes, stirring occasionally.

5. Stir the cooked lentils into the vegetable mixture. Transfer to a 9x13 inch baking dish.

6. In a large pot, cover the potato chunks with water and bring to a boil. Reduce heat and simmer for 15-20 minutes, until potatoes are very tender. Drain and return to the pot.

7. Mash the potatoes with the almond milk and olive oil. Season with salt and pepper.

8. Spread the mashed potatoes evenly over the lentil filling.

9. Bake for 30 minutes, until the potatoes are lightly browned on top.

10. Let stand for 5 minutes before serving.

This vegan shepherd's pie is packed with anti-inflammatory ingredients like lentils, vegetables, and potatoes. It's a comforting, nutrient-dense meal for seniors. Adjust seasoning to your taste preferences.

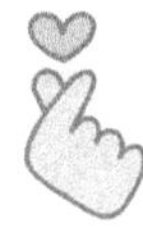

What are the critical points in the recipe (e.g., temperature control, timing)?

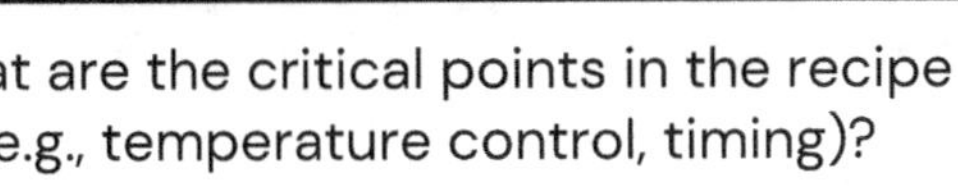

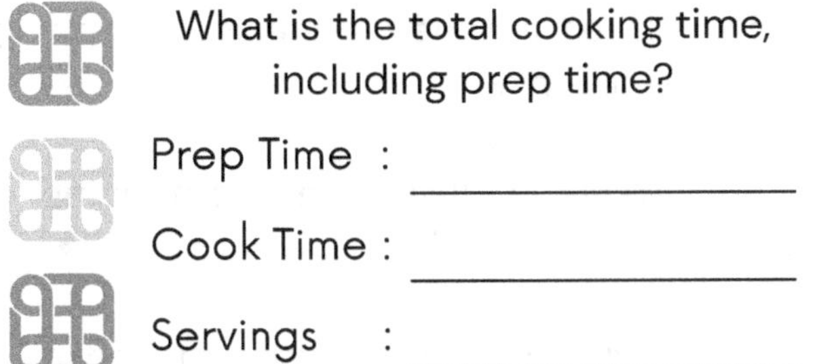
What is the total cooking time, including prep time?

Prep Time : _______________

Cook Time : _______________

Servings   : _______________

Ingredients:

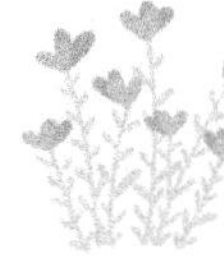

- 3 medium zucchini, spiralized or julienned into noodles
- 1/2 cup basil pesto (store-bought or homemade)
- 1 cup cherry tomatoes, halved
- 2 tablespoons toasted pine nuts
- 2 tablespoons grated Parmesan cheese (optional)
- Salt and pepper to taste

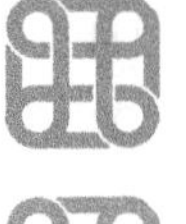
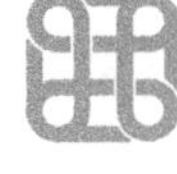
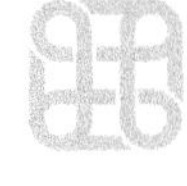
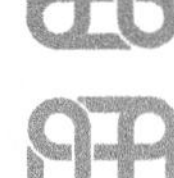

Is the recipe easy to follow?

40. Zucchini Noodles with Pesto and Cherry Tomatoes

1. In a large bowl, toss the zucchini noodles with the basil pesto until the noodles are evenly coated.

2. Add the halved cherry tomatoes and toss gently to combine.

3. Top the zucchini noodle mixture with the toasted pine nuts and grated Parmesan cheese (if using).

4. Season with salt and pepper to taste.

5. Serve immediately.

Tips:
- For a creamier texture, you can lightly sauté the zucchini noodles in a skillet with a bit of olive oil before tossing with the pesto.
- Customize the pesto by using different herbs, nuts, or cheeses.
- Add grilled chicken or shrimp for extra protein.
- Garnish with fresh basil leaves or a drizzle of balsamic glaze.

This dish is light, fresh, and packed with nutrients. The zucchini noodles provide a low-carb alternative to pasta, while the pesto, tomatoes, and pine nuts add flavor and healthy fats. It's a quick and easy meal that's perfect for a summer evening.

What are the critical points in the recipe (e.g., temperature control, timing)?

What is the total cooking time, including prep time?

Prep Time : _______________

Cook Time : _______________

Servings   : _______________

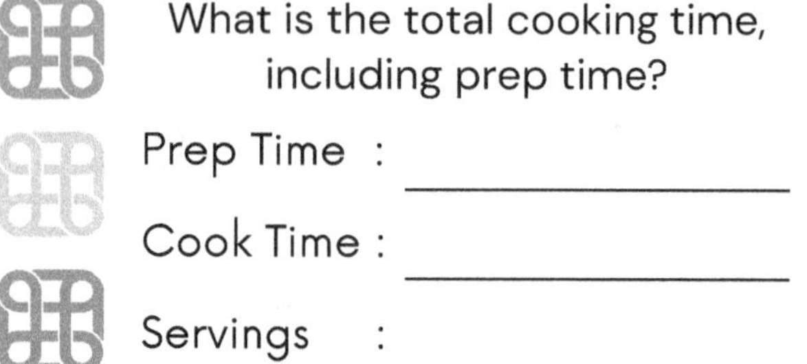

Ingredients:

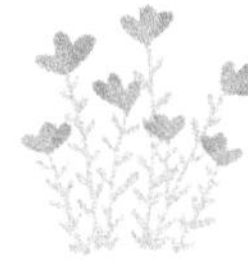

- 1/2 cup chia seeds
- 2 cups unsweetened almond milk
- 2 tablespoons maple syrup
- 1 teaspoon vanilla extract
- 1/4 teaspoon ground cinnamon
- 1 ripe mango, peeled and diced
- 1/4 cup unsweetened shredded coconut

1. In a medium bowl, whisk together the chia seeds, almond milk, maple syrup, vanilla, and cinnamon until well combined.

2. Cover the bowl and refrigerate for at least 4 hours, or overnight, stirring occasionally, until the chia seeds have thickened the mixture into a pudding-like consistency.

3. When ready to serve, divide the chia pudding evenly between 4 bowls or jars.

4. Top each serving with diced mango and a sprinkle of shredded coconut.

5. Serve chilled.

This chia pudding is packed with anti-inflammatory ingredients like chia seeds, mango, and coconut. The chia seeds provide fiber, protein, and omega-3s, while the mango offers vitamins, minerals, and antioxidants. The coconut adds healthy fats. It's a nourishing, refreshing dessert or snack for seniors.

You can adjust the sweetness by adding more or less maple syrup to your taste preferences. The chia pudding will keep refrigerated for up to 5 days, so it's a great make-ahead option.

Is the recipe easy to follow?

41. Chia Pudding with Mango and Coconut

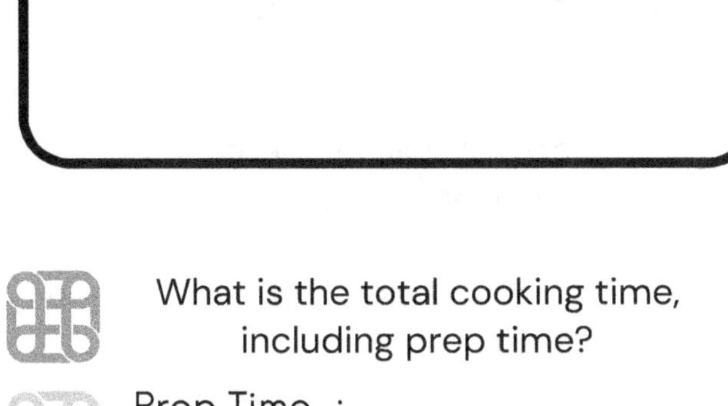

What are the critical points in the recipe (e.g., temperature control, timing)?

What is the total cooking time, including prep time?

Prep Time : _______________

Cook Time : _______________

Servings : _______________

Ingredients:

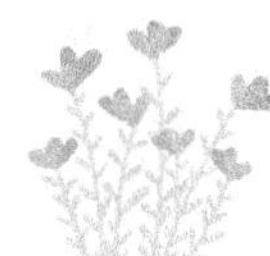

- 4 medium-sized apples (such as Honeycrisp or Gala)
- 1/4 cup chopped walnuts
- 2 tablespoons maple syrup
- 1 teaspoon ground cinnamon
- 1/4 teaspoon ground nutmeg
- 2 tablespoons unsweetened almond milk (or regular milk)
- Pinch of salt

Is the recipe easy to follow?

42. Baked Apples with Cinnamon and Walnuts

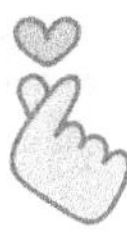

Procedure:

1. Preheat the oven to 375°F. Lightly grease a baking dish or line it with parchment paper.

2. Core the apples, leaving the bottom intact so they can stand upright. Use a paring knife or melon baller to scoop out the core, creating a well in the center of each apple.

3. In a small bowl, mix together the chopped walnuts, maple syrup, cinnamon, and nutmeg.

4. Stuff the walnut mixture into the center of each apple, packing it in tightly.

5. Place the stuffed apples in the prepared baking dish. Pour the almond milk around the base of the apples.

6. Bake for 30-40 minutes, until the apples are tender when pierced with a fork. Baste the apples with the liquid in the dish a few times during baking.

7. Remove from the oven and let cool for 5 minutes. Serve warm, with a sprinkle of salt over the top.

These baked apples are a delicious and anti-inflammatory dessert or snack for seniors. The walnuts provide healthy fats and antioxidants, while the cinnamon and nutmeg offer anti-inflammatory benefits. The maple syrup provides natural sweetness. Adjust the baking time as needed based on the size of your apples.

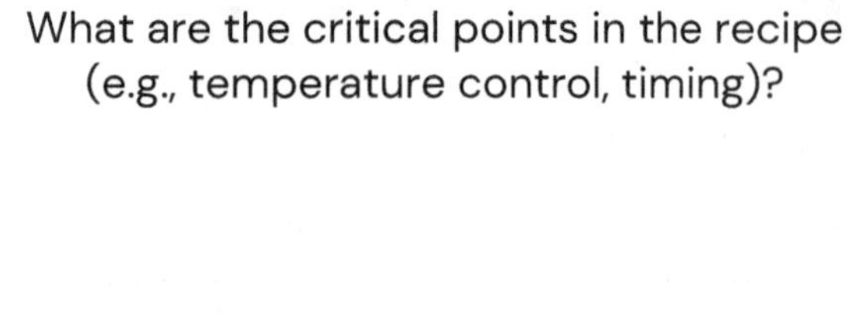

What are the critical points in the recipe (e.g., temperature control, timing)?

1. Break or chop the dark chocolate into small pieces.

2. Place the dark chocolate pieces and raw almonds in a small bowl or plate.

That's it! This is a quick and easy anti-inflammatory snack.

The benefits of this snack include:

Dark Chocolate:
- High in antioxidants that can help reduce inflammation
- Contains flavanols that may improve blood flow and lower blood pressure

Almonds:
- Rich in healthy monounsaturated fats, fiber, and antioxidants
- Provide anti-inflammatory magnesium, vitamin E, and other nutrients

Together, the dark chocolate and almonds make a delicious and satisfying snack that can help support an anti-inflammatory diet for seniors.

Some tips:
- Choose dark chocolate with 70% cacao or higher for maximum antioxidant benefits
- Opt for raw, unsalted almonds to avoid added oils and salt
- Portion the snack into small servings, as dark chocolate is high in calories
- Enjoy this snack in moderation as part of an overall healthy diet

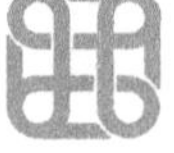

What is the total cooking time, including prep time?

Prep Time : _________________

Cook Time : _________________

Servings   : _________________

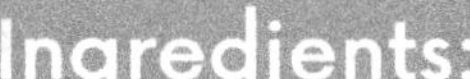 Ingredients: 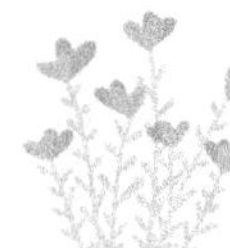

- 1 oz dark chocolate (70% cacao or higher)
- 1/4 cup raw, unsalted almonds

Is the recipe easy to follow?

😊   ☹️

43. Dark Chocolate with Almonds

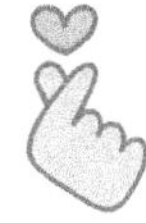

Procedure:

1. In a parfait glass or small bowl, layer half of the mixed berries on the bottom.

2. Top the berries with half of the coconut yogurt.

3. Repeat the layers of berries and yogurt.

4. Sprinkle the chopped toasted coconut over the top.

5. If desired, drizzle a small amount of honey over the parfait.

6. Serve chilled.

This parfait is a delicious and healthy treat that's perfect for any time of day. The benefits include:

- Mixed Berries: Packed with antioxidants, fiber, and vitamins to support overall health.

- Coconut Yogurt: Provides probiotics for gut health, as well as healthy fats from the coconut.

- Toasted Coconut: Adds a nice crunch and extra coconut flavor.

- Honey (optional): Adds a touch of natural sweetness.

The layered parfait looks beautiful and is easy to assemble. It's a refreshing and satisfying snack or light dessert. Adjust the amounts of each ingredient to suit your taste preferences. Enjoy!

What is the total cooking time, including prep time?

Prep Time : ________________

Cook Time : ________________

Servings   : ________________

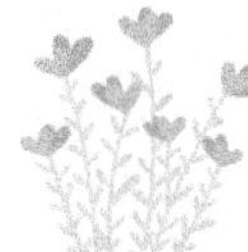

Ingredients:

- 1 cup mixed berries (such as raspberries, blueberries, and blackberries)
- 1 cup unsweetened coconut yogurt
- 2 tablespoons chopped toasted coconut
- 1 tablespoon honey (optional)

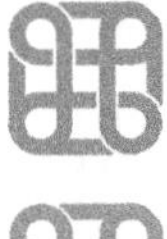
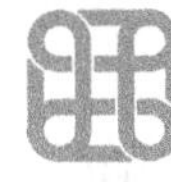
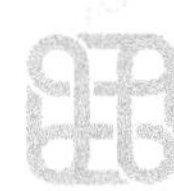
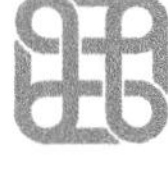
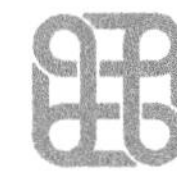

Is the recipe easy to follow?

44. Mixed Berry Parfait with Coconut Yogurt

What are the critical points in the recipe
(e.g., temperature control, timing)?

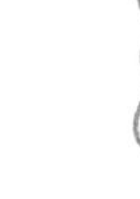

What is the total cooking time,
including prep time?

Prep Time : _________________

Cook Time : _________________

Servings : _________________

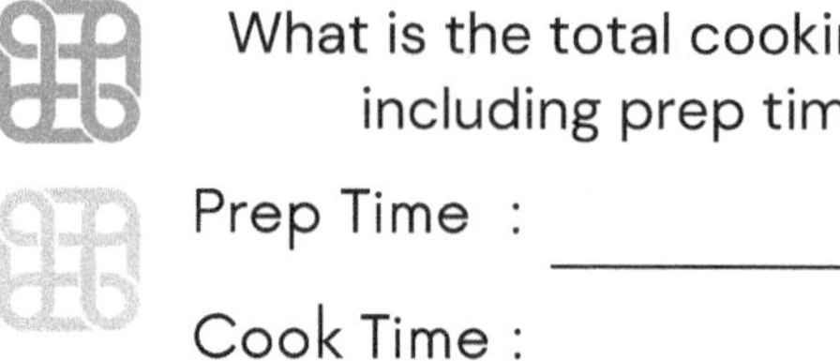

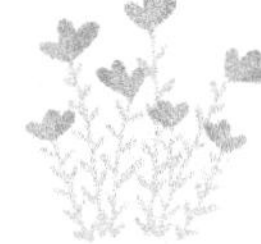

- 1 cup pitted Medjool dates
- 1/2 cup raw walnuts
- 1/2 cup raw almonds
- 2 tablespoons unsweetened shredded coconut
- 1 tablespoon ground flaxseed
- 1 teaspoon ground cinnamon
- 1/4 teaspoon ground ginger
- Pinch of sea salt

Is the recipe easy to follow?

45. Date and Nut Energy Balls

1. In a food processor, pulse the dates until they form a sticky paste.

2. Add the walnuts, almonds, coconut, flaxseed, cinnamon, ginger, and salt. Pulse until the mixture is well combined and starts to form a dough.

3. Scoop out tablespoon-sized portions of the mixture and roll them into balls with your hands.

4. Place the energy balls on a parchment-lined baking sheet and refrigerate for at least 30 minutes to firm up.

5. Store the energy balls in an airtight container in the refrigerator for up to 1 week.

These date and nut energy balls are packed with anti-inflammatory ingredients:

- Dates provide natural sweetness and fiber
- Walnuts and almonds are rich in healthy fats and antioxidants
- Coconut adds healthy fats
- Flaxseed is high in omega-3s
- Cinnamon and ginger have anti-inflammatory properties

They make a great snack or mini-meal for seniors, providing sustained energy and nutrition. Adjust the spices to your taste preferences. Enjoy!

What are the critical points in the recipe (e.g., temperature control, timing)?

What is the total cooking time, including prep time?

Prep Time : _______________

Cook Time : _______________

Servings   : _______________

Ingredients:

- 2 cups chopped fresh fruit (such as mango, pineapple, berries, or a mix)
- 2 tablespoons honey or maple syrup (optional)
- 1 tablespoon fresh lemon or lime juice

Is the recipe easy to follow?

😊 ☹️

46. Fresh Fruit Sorbet

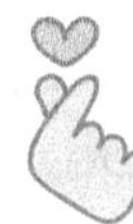

Procedure:

1. In a food processor or high-powered blender, puree the chopped fresh fruit until smooth.

2. If the fruit is not very sweet, add the honey or maple syrup and blend again until well incorporated.

3. Stir in the lemon or lime juice.

4. Pour the fruit puree into a shallow baking dish or metal pan and place in the freezer.

5. Every 30 minutes, use a fork to stir and scrape the partially frozen edges into the center. This will help create a smooth, sorbet-like texture.

6. Continue this process for 2-3 hours, until the sorbet Is completely frozen and scoopable.

7. Serve the fresh fruit sorbet immediately or transfer to an airtight container and freeze for up to 2 weeks.

This sorbet is a refreshing and anti-inflammatory treat for seniors. The fresh fruit provides vitamins, minerals, and antioxidants, while the optional honey or maple syrup adds natural sweetness. The citrus juice helps balance the flavors.

Some great fruit combinations to try:
- Mango and pineapple
- Strawberry and kiwi
- Blueberry and lemon
- Raspberry and blackberry

Adjust the sweetener to your taste preferences. Enjoy this healthy, homemade sorbet!

What are the critical points in the recipe (e.g., temperature control, timing)?

What is the total cooking time, including prep time?

Prep Time : _______________

Cook Time : _______________

Servings   : _______________

Ingredients:

- 1 cup almond flour
- 1/2 cup unsweetened shredded coconut
- 1/4 cup coconut oil, melted
- 2 tablespoons honey
- 1 teaspoon vanilla extract
- 1/4 teaspoon ground cinnamon
- 1/8 teaspoon sea salt

Is the recipe easy to follow?

47. Almond and Coconut Cookies

1. Preheat the oven to 325°F. Line a baking sheet with parchment paper.

2. In a medium bowl, stir together the almond flour and shredded coconut.

3. In a small bowl, whisk together the melted coconut oil, honey, vanilla, cinnamon, and salt.

4. Pour the wet ingredients into the dry ingredients and mix until a dough forms.

5. Scoop tablespoon-sized balls of dough and place them about 2 inches apart on the prepared baking sheet.

6. Gently flatten each cookie with the back of a fork.

7. Bake for 12-15 minutes, until the edges are lightly golden.

8. Allow the cookies to cool on the baking sheet for 5 minutes before transferring to a wire rack to cool completely.

These almond and coconut cookies are a delicious and anti-inflammatory treat for seniors. The almond flour and coconut provide healthy fats, while the honey adds natural sweetness. The cinnamon provides additional anti-inflammatory benefits.

Store the cookies in an airtight container at room temperature for up to 1 week. Enjoy these nutrient-dense cookies as a snack or light dessert.

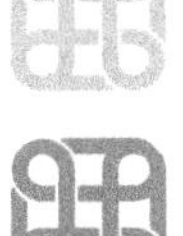

What is the total cooking time, including prep time?

Prep Time : ________________

Cook Time : ________________

Servings   : ________________

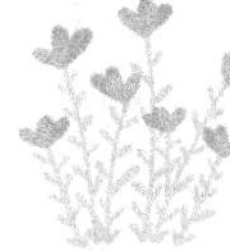

Ingredients:

For the Filling:
- 4 cups fresh or frozen blueberries
- 2 tablespoons honey
- 1 tablespoon lemon juice
- 1 teaspoon ground cinnamon
- 1/4 teaspoon ground ginger

For the Crumble Topping:
- 1 cup old-fashioned oats
- 1/2 cup almond flour
- 1/4 cup chopped walnuts
- 2 tablespoons coconut oil, melted
- 1 tablespoon honey
- 1/4 teaspoon ground cinnamon

Is the recipe easy to follow?

48. Blueberry and Oat Crumble

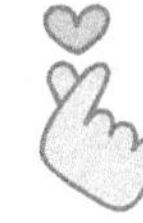

Procedure:

1. Preheat the oven to 375°F. Grease an 8x8 inch baking dish.

2. In a medium bowl, gently toss together the blueberries, honey, lemon juice, cinnamon, and ginger. Pour the filling into the prepared baking dish.

3. In a separate bowl, mix together the oats, almond flour, walnuts, melted coconut oil, honey, and cinnamon until well combined.

4. Sprinkle the oat crumble topping evenly over the blueberry filling.

5. Bake for 30-35 minutes, until the topping is golden brown and the filling is bubbling.

6. Allow the crumble to cool for 10-15 minutes before serving.

7. Serve warm, with a scoop of vanilla ice cream or a dollop of plain Greek yogurt, if desired.

This blueberry and oat crumble is packed with anti-inflammatory ingredients like blueberries, walnuts, and cinnamon. The oats and almond flour provide complex carbs and fiber, while the honey adds natural sweetness. It's a comforting and nutritious dessert or snack for seniors.

Adjust the sweetener and spices to your taste preferences. Enjoy this delicious and healthy crumble!

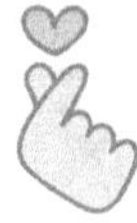

What is the total cooking time,
including prep time?

Prep Time : ___________________

Cook Time : ___________________

Servings   : ___________________

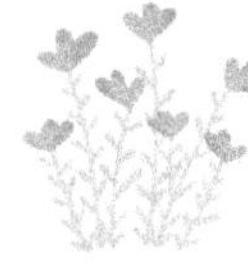

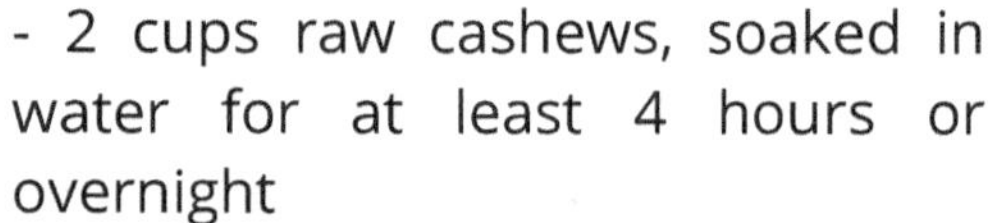

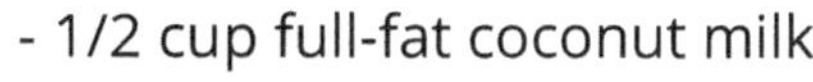

- 1 cup raw walnuts
- 1 cup raw almonds
- 1 cup pitted Medjool dates
- 1/4 teaspoon sea salt

Filling
- 2 cups raw cashews, soaked in water for at least 4 hours or overnight
- 1/2 cup full-fat coconut milk
- 1/4 cup maple syrup
- 2 tablespoons lemon juice
- 1 teaspoon vanilla extract
- 1/4 teaspoon sea salt

Is the recipe easy to follow?

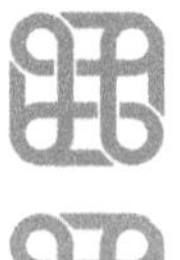

49. Raw Vegan Cheesecake

For the Crust:
1. In a food processor, pulse the walnuts, almonds, dates, and salt until the mixture sticks together when pressed.
2. Press the crust mixture evenly into the bottom of a 9-inch springform pan. Refrigerate while making the filling.

For the Filling:
1. Drain and rinse the soaked cashews. Add them to a high-speed blender along with the coconut milk, maple syrup, lemon juice, vanilla, and salt.
2. Blend on high speed until the mixture is completely smooth and creamy, about 2-3 minutes.
3. Pour the filling over the chilled crust and smooth the top.
4. Refrigerate the cheesecake for at least 4 hours, or until set.

To Serve:
1. Release the springform pan and slice the cheesecake.
2. Top with fresh berries, a drizzle of maple syrup, or a sprinkle of toasted coconut, if desired.

This raw vegan cheesecake is packed with anti-inflammatory ingredients like nuts, coconut, and lemon. The cashews provide a creamy texture without dairy. It's a delicious and nutritious dessert that's perfect for seniors. Adjust the sweetness to your taste preferences.

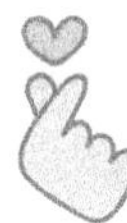

Procedure:

1. In a high-powered blender or food processor, blend the frozen bananas until smooth and creamy, scraping down the sides as needed.

2. Add the frozen mixed berries, almond milk, vanilla extract, and cinnamon. Blend again until well combined and the berries are broken down.

3. Serve the banana ice cream immediately, or transfer to an airtight container and freeze for 1-2 hours for a firmer consistency.

4. Scoop the banana ice cream into bowls and top with any additional fresh or frozen berries, if desired.

This banana ice cream is a delicious and anti-inflammatory treat for seniors. The benefits include:

- Bananas: Provide potassium, fiber, and natural sweetness.
- Berries: Rich in antioxidants, vitamins, and anti-inflammatory compounds.
- Cinnamon: Has anti-inflammatory properties.
- Almond milk: Adds creaminess without dairy.

The frozen bananas create a creamy, ice cream-like texture without the need for any added sugars or heavy cream. It's a refreshing and nutritious dessert or snack.

You can experiment with different berry combinations or add a drizzle of honey for extra sweetness. Enjoy this healthy banana ice cream!

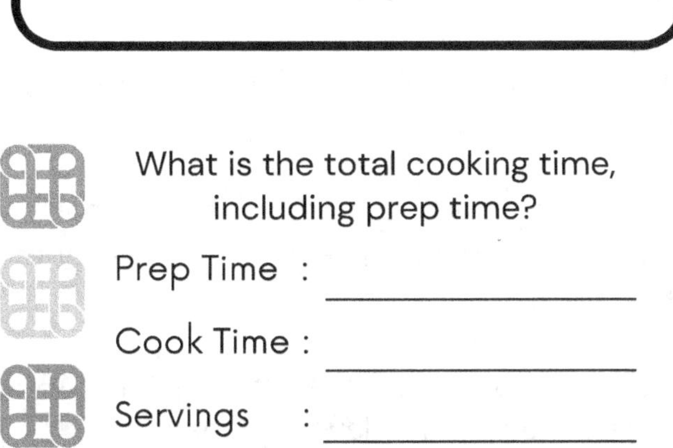

What is the total cooking time, including prep time?

Prep Time : _________________

Cook Time : _________________

Servings : _________________

Ingredients:

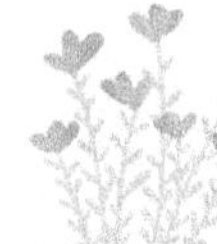

- 3 ripe bananas, peeled and frozen
- 1/2 cup frozen mixed berries (such as raspberries, blueberries, and blackberries)
- 1 tablespoon almond milk (or regular milk)
- 1 teaspoon vanilla extract
- 1/4 teaspoon ground cinnamon

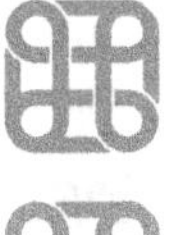
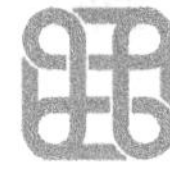
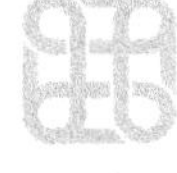
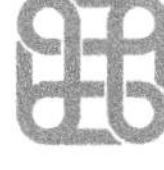
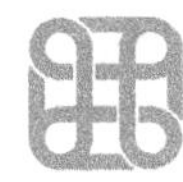

Is the recipe easy to follow?

50. Banana Ice Cream with Berries

Procedure:

What is the total cooking time,
including prep time?

Prep Time : ___________________

Cook Time : ___________________

Servings   : ___________________

Ingredients:

- 2 tablespoons olive oil
- 1 onion, diced
- 3 cloves garlic, minced
- 2 (28 oz) cans diced tomatoes
- 2 cups low-sodium vegetable or chicken broth
- 1/4 cup fresh basil leaves, chopped
- 1 teaspoon dried oregano
- 1/2 teaspoon ground cumin
- Salt and pepper to taste
- Grated Parmesan cheese for serving (optional)

Is the recipe easy to follow?

51. Tomato and Basil Soup

1. In a large pot or Dutch oven, heat the olive oil over medium heat. Add the onion and sauté for 5 minutes until translucent.

2. Add the garlic and cook for 1 minute, stirring constantly, until fragrant.

3. Stir in the diced tomatoes, broth, basil, oregano, and cumin. Season with salt and pepper.

4. Bring the soup to a simmer and cook for 15-20 minutes, allowing the flavors to meld.

5. Using an immersion blender, carefully puree the soup until smooth. Alternatively, you can transfer the soup in batches to a regular blender.

6. Taste and adjust seasoning as needed.

7. Ladle the tomato and basil soup into bowls and garnish with grated Parmesan cheese, if desired.

This creamy, flavorful soup is packed with anti-inflammatory ingredients. Tomatoes are rich in lycopene, while fresh basil provides antioxidants and anti-inflammatory properties. The warming spices add depth of flavor.

It's a comforting and nourishing soup that's perfect for seniors. Adjust the consistency by adding more or less broth to your desired thickness. Enjoy this delicious and healthy soup!

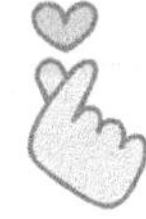

Procedure:

What is the total cooking time, including prep time?

Prep Time : ___________________

Cook Time : ___________________

Servings : ___________________

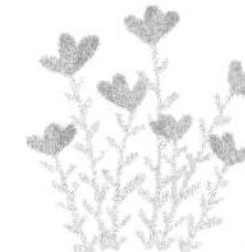

Ingredients:

- 1 medium butternut squash, peeled, seeded, and cubed (about 4 cups)
- 1 tablespoon olive oil
- 1 onion, diced
- 3 cloves garlic, minced
- 2 tablespoons grated fresh ginger
- 4 cups low-sodium vegetable or chicken broth
- 1 teaspoon ground cumin
- 1/2 teaspoon ground cinnamon
- Salt and pepper to taste
- Chopped fresh parsley for garnish

1. In a large pot or Dutch oven, heat the olive oil over medium heat. Add the onion and sauté for 5 minutes until translucent.

2. Add the garlic and grated ginger. Cook for 1 minute, stirring constantly, until fragrant.

3. Stir in the cubed butternut squash, broth, cumin, and cinnamon. Season with salt and pepper.

4. Bring the soup to a boil, then reduce heat and simmer for 20-25 minutes, until the squash is very tender.

5. Using an immersion blender, carefully puree the soup until smooth. Alternatively, you can transfer the soup in batches to a regular blender.

6. Taste and adjust seasoning as needed.

7. Ladle the butternut squash soup into bowls and garnish with chopped fresh parsley.

This creamy, flavorful soup is packed with anti-inflammatory ingredients. Butternut squash is high in beta-carotene, while ginger provides natural anti-inflammatory properties. The warming spices add depth of flavor. It's a comforting and nourishing soup that's perfect for seniors.

You can adjust the consistency of the soup by adding more or less broth to your desired thickness. Enjoy this delicious and healthy soup!

Is the recipe easy to follow?

52. Butternut Squash Soup with Ginger

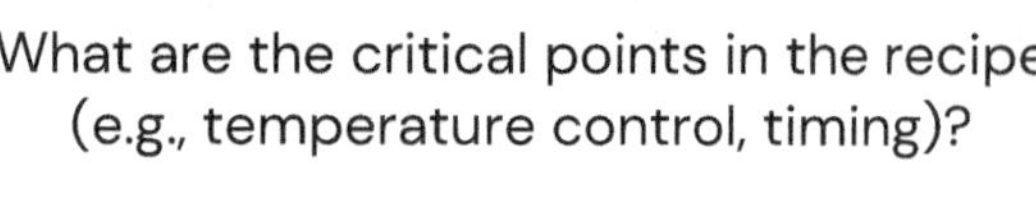

What are the critical points in the recipe (e.g., temperature control, timing)?

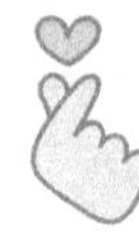

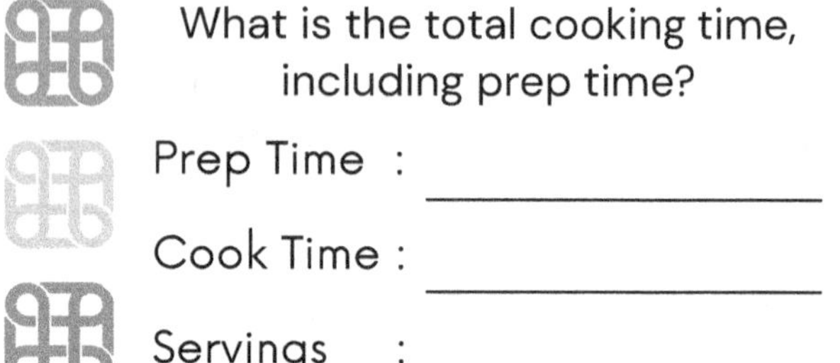

What is the total cooking time, including prep time?

Prep Time : ______________

Cook Time : ______________

Servings   : ______________

Ingredients:

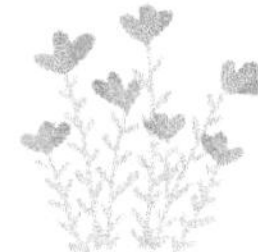

- 1 tablespoon olive oil
- 1 onion, diced
- 3 cloves garlic, minced
- 1 tablespoon grated fresh ginger
- 1 cup red lentils, rinsed
- 4 cups low-sodium vegetable or chicken broth
- 3 carrots, peeled and sliced
- 1 teaspoon ground cumin
- 1/2 teaspoon ground coriander
- 1/4 teaspoon ground turmeric
- Salt and pepper to taste
- Chopped fresh cilantro for garnish

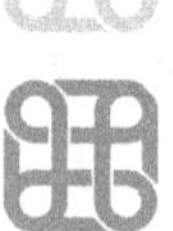

Is the recipe easy to follow?

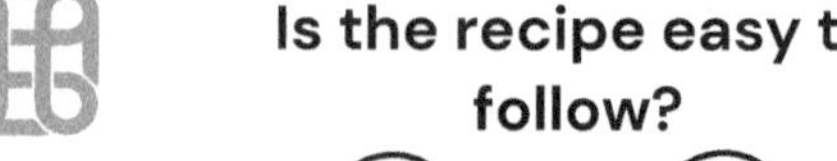

53. *Red Lentil Soup with Carrots*

1. In a large pot or Dutch oven, heat the olive oil over medium heat. Add the onion and sauté for 5 minutes until translucent.

2. Add the garlic and grated ginger. Cook for 1 minute, stirring constantly, until fragrant.

3. Stir in the rinsed red lentils, broth, sliced carrots, cumin, coriander, and turmeric. Season with salt and pepper.

4. Bring the soup to a boil, then reduce heat and simmer for 20-25 minutes, until the lentils and carrots are very tender.

5. Using an immersion blender, carefully puree the soup until smooth. Alternatively, you can transfer the soup in batches to a regular blender.

6. Taste and adjust seasoning as needed.

7. Ladle the red lentil soup into bowls and garnish with chopped fresh cilantro.

This creamy, nourishing soup is packed with anti-inflammatory ingredients. The red lentils provide protein and fiber, while the carrots, ginger, and spices offer additional anti-inflammatory benefits. It's a comforting and easy-to-digest meal for seniors.

Adjust the consistency of the soup by adding more or less broth to your desired thickness. Enjoy this delicious and healthy red lentil soup!

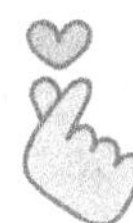

What are the critical points in the recipe (e.g., temperature control, timing)?

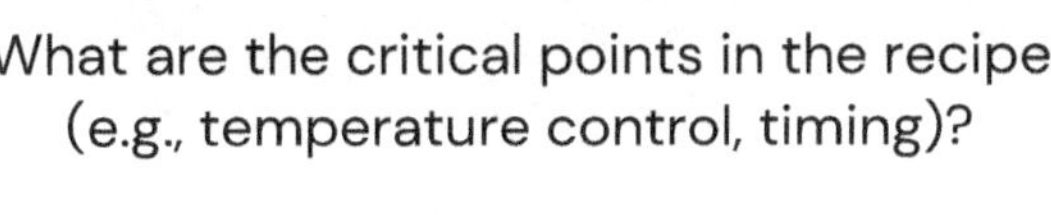

What is the total cooking time, including prep time?

Prep Time : ________________

Cook Time : ________________

Servings   : ________________

Ingredients:

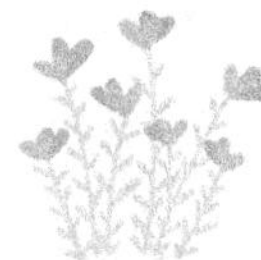

- 1 tablespoon olive oil
- 1 onion, diced
- 3 cloves garlic, minced
- 2 carrots, peeled and diced
- 2 stalks celery, diced
- 1 cup pearl barley, rinsed
- 4 cups low-sodium vegetable or chicken broth
- 1 (14 oz) can diced tomatoes
- 1 bay leaf
- 1 teaspoon dried thyme
- 1/2 teaspoon ground cumin
- Salt and pepper to taste
- 2 cups chopped kale or spinach
- 2 tablespoons chopped fresh parsley

Is the recipe easy to follow?

54. Vegetable and Barley Stew

1. In a large pot or Dutch oven, heat the olive oil over medium heat. Add the onion and sauté for 5 minutes until translucent.

2. Add the garlic, carrots, and celery. Cook for 3-4 minutes, stirring frequently, until the vegetables start to soften.

3. Stir in the rinsed barley, broth, diced tomatoes, bay leaf, thyme, and cumin. Season with salt and pepper.

4. Bring the stew to a boil, then reduce heat and simmer for 30-35 minutes, until the barley is tender.

5. Remove the bay leaf. Stir in the chopped kale or spinach and cook for 2-3 minutes until wilted.

6. Taste and adjust seasoning as needed.

7. Ladle the vegetable and barley stew into bowls and garnish with chopped fresh parsley.

This hearty stew is packed with anti-inflammatory ingredients like vegetables, barley, and leafy greens. The fiber, complex carbs, and nutrients make it a nourishing and satisfying meal for seniors. Adjust the vegetables and seasonings to your taste preferences.

The barley provides a creamy, comforting texture, while the kale or spinach adds extra vitamins and minerals. Enjoy this delicious and healthy stew!

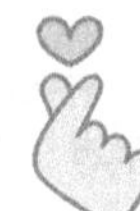

Procedure:

1. In a large pot or Dutch oven, heat the olive oil over medium heat. Add the onion and sauté for 5 minutes until translucent.

2. Add the garlic and mushrooms. Cook for 5-7 minutes, stirring occasionally, until the mushrooms are tender.

3. Stir in the uncooked wild rice blend, broth, almond milk, thyme, and sage. Season with salt and pepper.

4. Bring the soup to a boil, then reduce heat and simmer for 40-45 minutes, until the rice is tender.

5. Taste and adjust seasoning as needed.

6. Ladle the mushroom and wild rice soup into bowls and garnish with chopped fresh parsley.

This creamy, earthy soup is packed with anti-inflammatory ingredients. The mushrooms provide antioxidants, while the wild rice offers complex carbs, fiber, and nutrients. The almond milk adds creaminess without dairy.

The warming spices like thyme and sage complement the mushroom flavor. It's a comforting and nourishing soup that's perfect for seniors. Adjust the consistency by adding more or less broth to your desired thickness. Enjoy this delicious and healthy soup!

What is the total cooking time, including prep time?

Prep Time : _________________

Cook Time : _________________

Servings   : _________________

Ingredients:

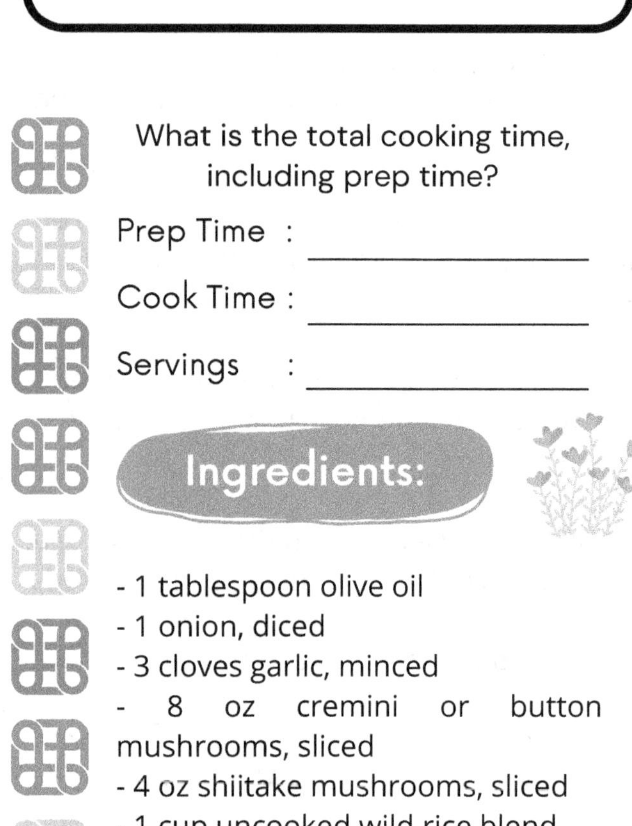

- 1 tablespoon olive oil
- 1 onion, diced
- 3 cloves garlic, minced
- 8 oz cremini or button mushrooms, sliced
- 4 oz shiitake mushrooms, sliced
- 1 cup uncooked wild rice blend
- 4 cups low-sodium vegetable or chicken broth
- 2 cups unsweetened almond milk
- 1 teaspoon dried thyme
- 1/2 teaspoon ground sage
- Salt and pepper to taste
- Chopped fresh parsley for garnish

Is the recipe easy to follow?

55. *Mushroom and Wild Rice Soup*

What are the critical points in the recipe (e.g., temperature control, timing)?

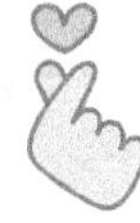

What is the total cooking time, including prep time?

Prep Time : _________________

Cook Time : _________________

Servings   : _________________

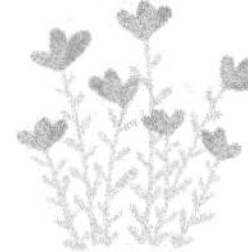

Ingredients:

- 1 tablespoon olive oil
- 1 onion, diced
- 3 cloves garlic, minced
- 1 tablespoon grated fresh ginger
- 1 lb carrots, peeled and sliced
- 4 cups low-sodium vegetable or chicken broth
- 1 teaspoon ground cumin
- 1/2 teaspoon ground coriander
- Salt and pepper to taste
- Chopped fresh parsley for garnish

Is the recipe easy to follow?

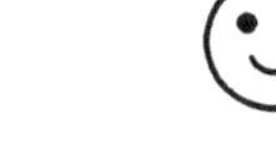

56. Carrot and Ginger Soup

1. In a large pot or Dutch oven, heat the olive oil over medium heat. Add the onion and sauté for 5 minutes until translucent.

2. Add the garlic and grated ginger. Cook for 1 minute, stirring constantly, until fragrant.

3. Stir in the sliced carrots, broth, cumin, and coriander. Season with salt and pepper.

4. Bring the soup to a boil, then reduce heat and simmer for 20-25 minutes, until the carrots are very tender.

5. Using an immersion blender, carefully puree the soup until smooth. Alternatively, you can transfer the soup in batches to a regular blender.

6. Taste and adjust seasoning as needed.

7. Ladle the carrot ginger soup into bowls and garnish with chopped fresh parsley.

This creamy carrot and ginger soup is packed with anti-inflammatory ingredients. The carrots are high in beta-carotene, while the ginger provides natural anti-inflammatory properties. It's a nourishing and comforting soup that's easy to digest for seniors. Adjust the spices to your taste preferences.

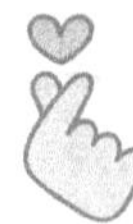

What is the total cooking time, including prep time?

Prep Time : _________________

Cook Time : _________________

Servings   : _________________

Ingredients:

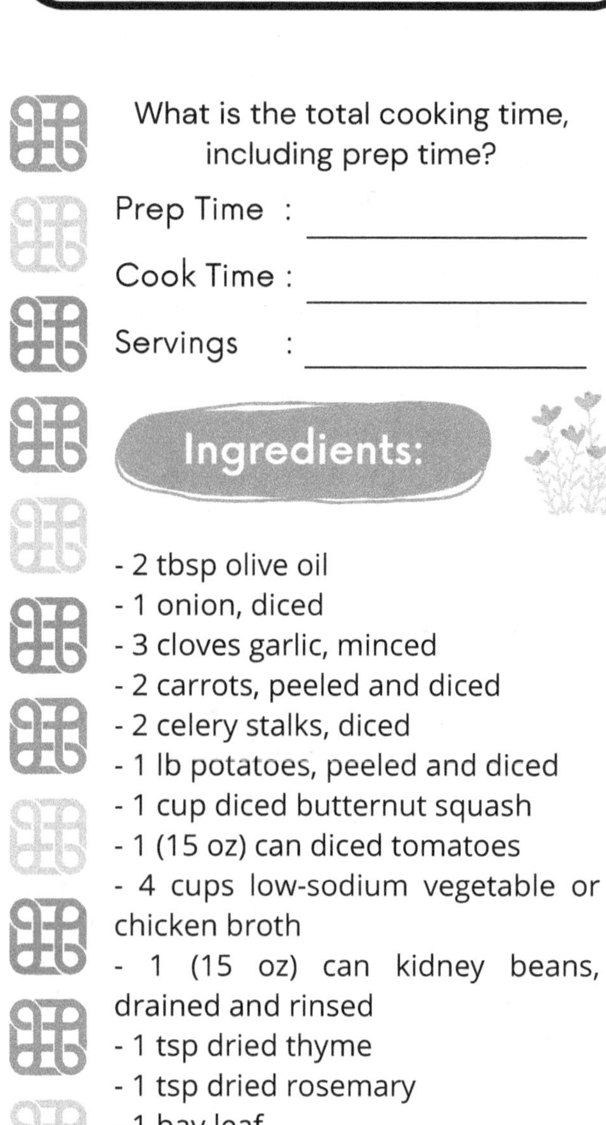

- 2 tbsp olive oil
- 1 onion, diced
- 3 cloves garlic, minced
- 2 carrots, peeled and diced
- 2 celery stalks, diced
- 1 lb potatoes, peeled and diced
- 1 cup diced butternut squash
- 1 (15 oz) can diced tomatoes
- 4 cups low-sodium vegetable or chicken broth
- 1 (15 oz) can kidney beans, drained and rinsed
- 1 tsp dried thyme
- 1 tsp dried rosemary
- 1 bay leaf
- Salt and pepper to taste
- Chopped parsley for garnish

Is the recipe easy to follow?

57. Hearty Vegetable Stew

1. In a large pot or Dutch oven, heat the olive oil over medium heat. Add the onion and sauté for 5 minutes until translucent.

2. Add the garlic, carrots, celery, potatoes and butternut squash. Cook for 5 more minutes, stirring occasionally.

3. Pour in the diced tomatoes, broth, kidney beans, thyme, rosemary and bay leaf. Season with salt and pepper.

4. Bring the stew to a boil, then reduce heat and simmer for 30-40 minutes, until the vegetables are very tender.

5. Remove the bay leaf. Taste and adjust seasonings as needed.

6. Serve the stew hot, garnished with chopped parsley.

This hearty vegetable stew is packed with anti-inflammatory ingredients like vegetables, beans, and herbs. The combination of nutrients can help reduce inflammation and support overall health, especially for seniors. The tender vegetables and broth-based preparation also make it an easy-to-digest meal.

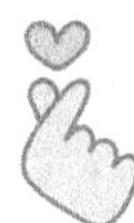

What are the critical points in the recipe (e.g., temperature control, timing)?

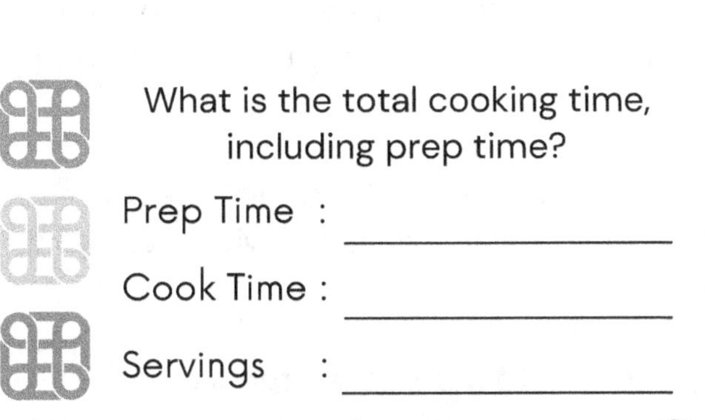

What is the total cooking time, including prep time?

Prep Time : ______________

Cook Time : ______________

Servings   : ______________

Ingredients:

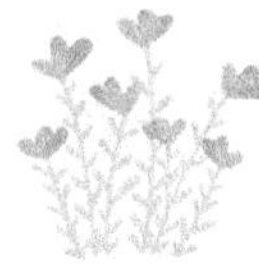

- 2 tbsp olive oil
- 1 onion, diced
- 3 cloves garlic, minced
- 1 tsp ground cumin
- 1 tsp ground coriander
- 1/4 tsp cayenne pepper (optional, for heat)
- 1 (15 oz) can pumpkin puree
- 1 (13.5 oz) can full-fat coconut milk
- 3 cups low-sodium vegetable or chicken broth
- 1 tsp salt
- 1/4 tsp black pepper
- Chopped cilantro for garnish

Is the recipe easy to follow?

58. *Pumpkin Soup with Coconut Milk*

1. In a large pot or Dutch oven, heat the olive oil over medium heat. Add the onion and sauté for 5 minutes until translucent.

2. Add the garlic, cumin, coriander and cayenne (if using). Cook for 1 minute until fragrant.

3. Stir in the pumpkin puree, coconut milk and broth. Season with salt and pepper.

4. Bring the soup to a simmer and cook for 15-20 minutes, stirring occasionally, until heated through.

5. Use an immersion blender to puree the soup until smooth (or carefully transfer to a blender in batches).

6. Taste and adjust seasonings as needed.

7. Serve the pumpkin soup hot, garnished with chopped cilantro.

This creamy pumpkin soup gets a boost of richness and creaminess from the addition of coconut milk. The warming spices like cumin and coriander complement the pumpkin flavor. It's a comforting, nourishing soup that's perfect for cool weather.

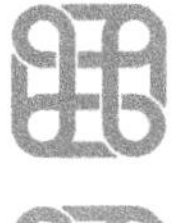

What is the total cooking time, including prep time?

Prep Time : _________________

Cook Time : _________________

Servings   : _________________

Ingredients:

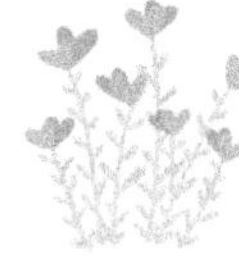

- 1 tbsp olive oil
- 1 onion, diced
- 3 cloves garlic, minced
- 2 tsp chili powder
- 1 tsp ground cumin
- 1 tsp dried oregano
- 1/4 tsp cayenne pepper (optional, for heat)
- 1 (15 oz) can black beans, drained and rinsed
- 1 (15 oz) can diced tomatoes
- 1 lb sweet potatoes, peeled and diced
- 2 cups vegetable or chicken broth
- Salt and pepper to taste
- Toppings: avocado, cilantro, sour cream, shredded cheese

Is the recipe easy to follow?

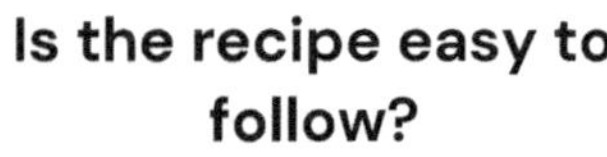

59. *Sweet Potato and Black Bean Chili*

1. In a large pot or Dutch oven, heat the olive oil over medium heat. Add the onion and sauté for 5 minutes until translucent.

2. Add the garlic, chili powder, cumin, oregano and cayenne (if using). Cook for 1 minute until fragrant.

3. Stir in the black beans, diced tomatoes, sweet potatoes and broth. Season with salt and pepper.

4. Bring the chili to a boil, then reduce heat and simmer for 20-25 minutes, until the sweet potatoes are tender.

5. Taste and adjust seasonings as needed.

6. Serve the chili hot, topped with desired toppings like avocado, cilantro, sour cream and shredded cheese.

Enjoy this hearty, vegetarian chili! The sweet potatoes and black beans make it a nutritious and filling meal.

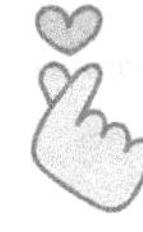

Procedure:

1. In a large pot or Dutch oven, heat the olive oil over medium heat. Add the onion and sauté for 5 minutes until translucent.

2. Add the garlic and cook for 1 minute until fragrant.

3. Stir in the diced zucchini and broth. Bring to a simmer.

4. Add the basil, oregano, cumin and cayenne (if using). Simmer for 15-20 minutes, until the zucchini is very tender.

5. Remove from heat and use an immersion blender to puree the soup until smooth (or carefully transfer to a blender in batches).

6. Stir in the white beans and season with salt and pepper to taste.

7. Serve the zucchini basil soup hot, with lemon wedges on the side.

This vibrant green soup is packed with anti-inflammatory ingredients like zucchini, basil, and white beans. The blend of aromatic herbs and spices adds great flavor while also providing antioxidant and anti-inflammatory benefits. The creamy texture and easy-to-digest ingredients make this an ideal soup for seniors.

What is the total cooking time, including prep time?

Prep Time : _________________

Cook Time : _________________

Servings : _________________

Ingredients:

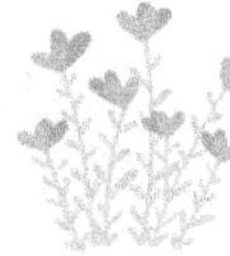

- 2 tbsp olive oil
- 1 onion, diced
- 3 cloves garlic, minced
- 2 lbs zucchini, diced
- 4 cups low-sodium vegetable or chicken broth
- 1 cup packed fresh basil leaves
- 1 tsp dried oregano
- 1 tsp ground cumin
- 1/4 tsp cayenne pepper (optional, for heat)
- 1 (15 oz) can white beans, drained and rinsed
- Salt and pepper to taste
- Lemon wedges for serving

Is the recipe easy to follow?

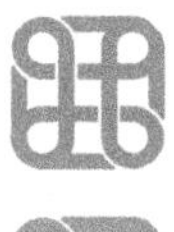
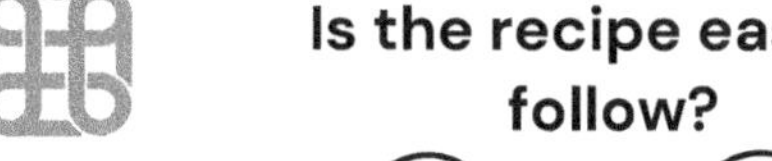

60. Zucchini and Basil Soup

Procedure:

1. In a large bowl, combine the chopped kale.

2. In a small bowl, whisk together the olive oil, lemon juice, Dijon mustard, garlic, and honey. Season with salt and pepper.

3. Pour the dressing over the kale and toss to coat evenly.

4. Top the salad with the diced avocado.

This salad is a great source of anti-inflammatory nutrients:

- Kale is high in antioxidants and vitamins A, C, and K, which can help reduce inflammation.

- Avocado is rich in healthy monounsaturated fats, vitamin E, and carotenoids that have anti-inflammatory properties.

- The lemon juice and Dijon mustard in the dressing provide additional anti-inflammatory benefits.

The healthy fats, vitamins, and antioxidants in this salad make it a great option for seniors looking to support their overall health and reduce inflammation.

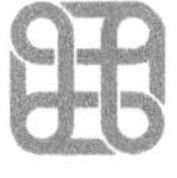

What is the total cooking time, including prep time?

Prep Time : ___________________

Cook Time : ___________________

Servings   : ___________________

Ingredients:

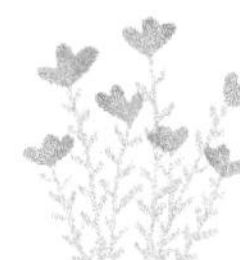

- 1 bunch kale, stems removed and leaves chopped
- 1 avocado, diced
- 1/4 cup olive oil
- 2 tbsp lemon juice
- 1 tbsp Dijon mustard
- 1 garlic clove, minced
- 1 tsp honey
- Salt and pepper to taste

Is the recipe easy to follow?

61. Kale Salad with Avocado and Lemon Dressing

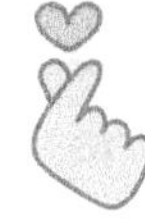

Procedure:

1. In a large salad bowl, combine the arugula, roasted beet slices, feta cheese and walnuts.

2. In a small bowl, whisk together the olive oil, balsamic vinegar, Dijon mustard and honey. Season with salt and pepper.

3. Drizzle the dressing over the salad and toss gently to coat.

4. Serve the arugula salad immediately.

This salad is packed with anti-inflammatory ingredients:

- Arugula is a nutrient-dense leafy green with antioxidants and anti-inflammatory properties.

- Beets are rich in betalains, which have potent anti-inflammatory effects.

- Walnuts contain omega-3 fatty acids that help reduce inflammation.

- Feta cheese provides protein and calcium.

The bright, tangy dressing complements the earthy flavors of the beets and the peppery arugula. This salad is easy to prepare and makes a great light meal or side dish for seniors. The combination of nutrients supports overall health and can help reduce inflammation.

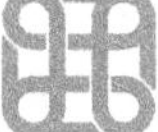

What is the total cooking time, including prep time?

Prep Time : _______________

Cook Time : _______________

Servings   : _______________

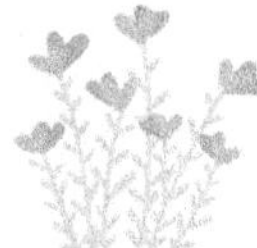

Ingredients:

- 5 oz baby arugula
- 2 medium beets, roasted, peeled and sliced
- 1/2 cup crumbled feta cheese
- 1/4 cup chopped walnuts
- 2 tbsp olive oil
- 1 tbsp balsamic vinegar
- 1 tsp Dijon mustard
- 1 tsp honey
- Salt and pepper to taste

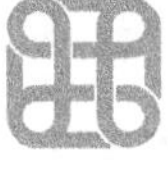
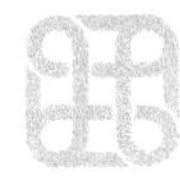
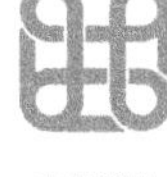
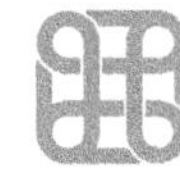

Is the recipe easy to follow?

62. Arugula Salad with Beets and Walnuts

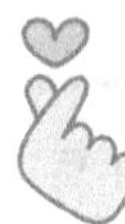

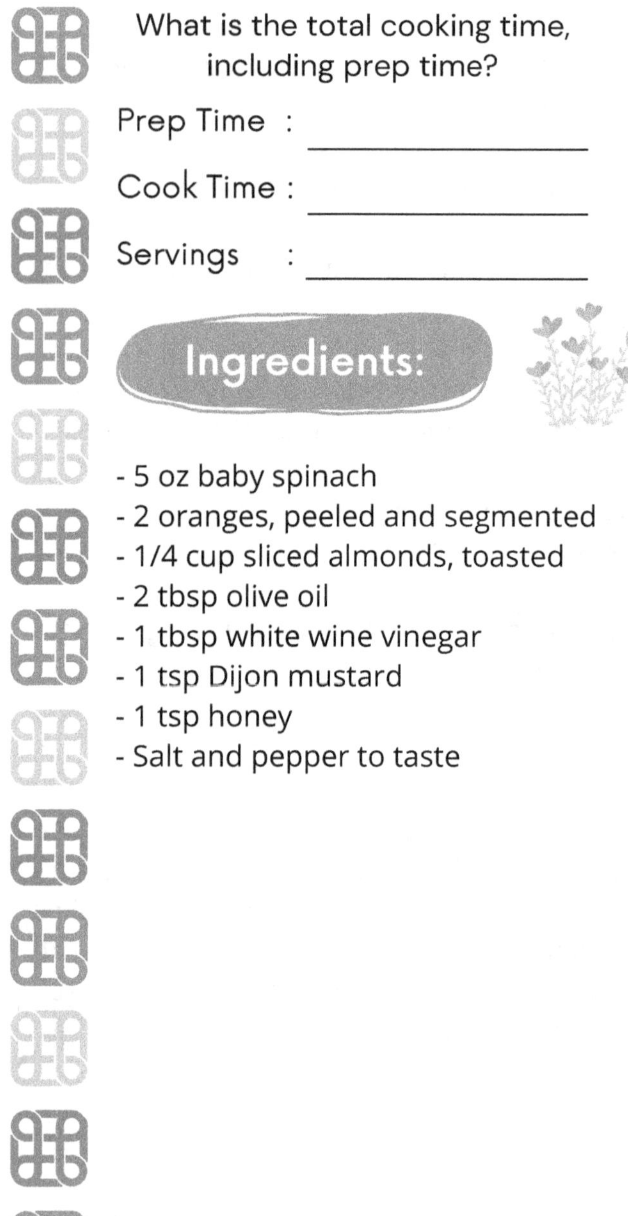

What is the total cooking time,
including prep time?

Prep Time : _______________

Cook Time : _______________

Servings   : _______________

Ingredients:

- 5 oz baby spinach
- 2 oranges, peeled and segmented
- 1/4 cup sliced almonds, toasted
- 2 tbsp olive oil
- 1 tbsp white wine vinegar
- 1 tsp Dijon mustard
- 1 tsp honey
- Salt and pepper to taste

**Is the recipe easy to
follow?**

63. Spinach Salad with Oranges and Almonds

1. In a large salad bowl, combine the baby spinach, orange segments and toasted almond slices.

2. In a small bowl, whisk together the olive oil, white wine vinegar, Dijon mustard and honey. Season with salt and pepper.

3. Drizzle the dressing over the spinach salad and toss gently to coat.

4. Serve the salad immediately.

This spinach salad is a delicious and nutritious option:

- Spinach is packed with vitamins, minerals and antioxidants that have anti-inflammatory properties.
- Oranges are high in vitamin C, which is a powerful antioxidant.
- Almonds provide healthy fats, protein and fiber.

The bright citrus flavors from the oranges pair beautifully with the earthy spinach and crunchy almonds. The light, tangy dressing ties all the flavors together.

This salad makes a great light meal or side dish. It's easy to prepare and the combination of nutrients makes it a healthy choice, especially for seniors looking to reduce inflammation.

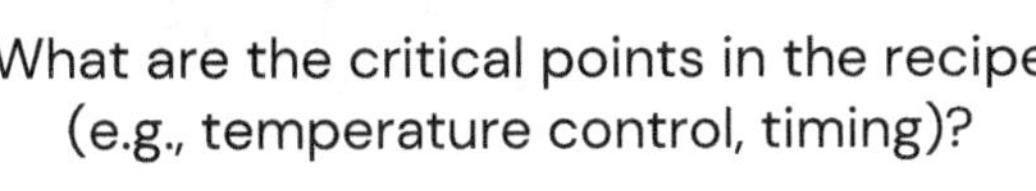

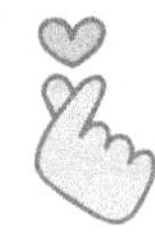

> What are the critical points in the recipe (e.g., temperature control, timing)?

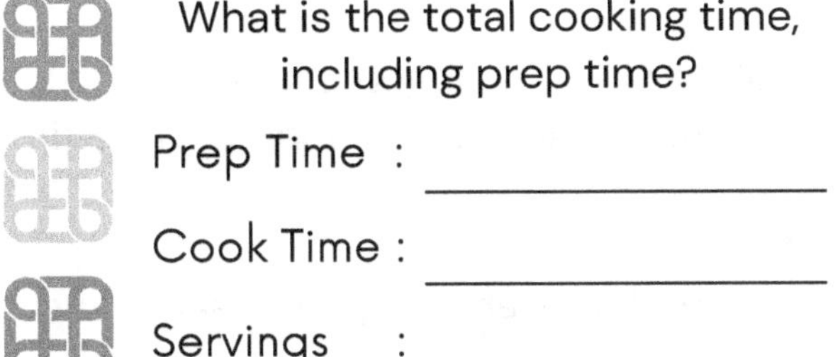

What is the total cooking time, including prep time?

Prep Time : _________________

Cook Time : _________________

Servings   : _________________

Ingredients:

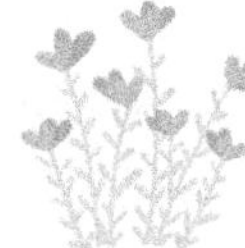

- 5 oz mixed greens (such as spinach, arugula, kale)
- 1/2 cup pomegranate seeds
- 1/4 cup crumbled feta cheese
- 2 tbsp toasted pumpkin seeds
- 2 tbsp olive oil
- 1 tbsp balsamic vinegar
- 1 tsp Dijon mustard
- 1 tsp honey
- Salt and pepper to taste

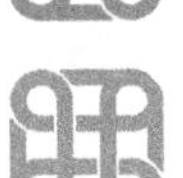
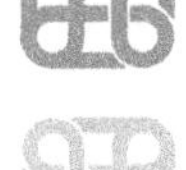
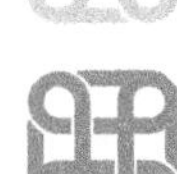
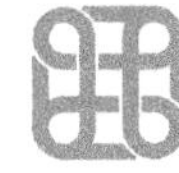
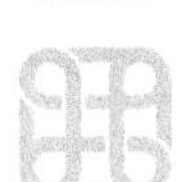

Is the recipe easy to follow?

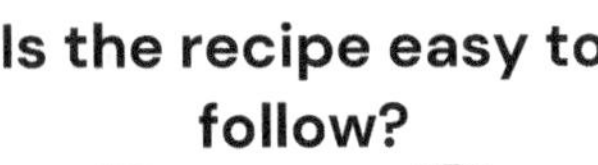

64. Mixed Green Salad with Pomegranate Seeds

Procedure:

1. In a large salad bowl, combine the mixed greens, pomegranate seeds, feta cheese and toasted pumpkin seeds.

2. In a small bowl, whisk together the olive oil, balsamic vinegar, Dijon mustard and honey. Season with salt and pepper.

3. Drizzle the dressing over the salad and toss gently to coat.

4. Serve the salad immediately.

This mixed green salad is a nutritious and flavorful option:

- The mixed greens provide a variety of vitamins, minerals and antioxidants.
- Pomegranate seeds are rich in polyphenols, which have potent anti-inflammatory properties.
- Feta cheese adds protein and calcium.
- Pumpkin seeds contain healthy fats, protein and magnesium.

The sweet-tart pomegranate seeds, salty feta, and crunchy pumpkin seeds create a delightful contrast of flavors and textures. The simple balsamic vinaigrette ties it all together.

This salad makes a great light meal or side dish. It's easy to prepare and the combination of nutrient-dense ingredients makes it a healthy choice, especially for seniors looking to reduce inflammation.

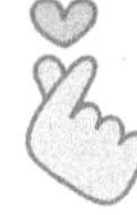

Procedure:

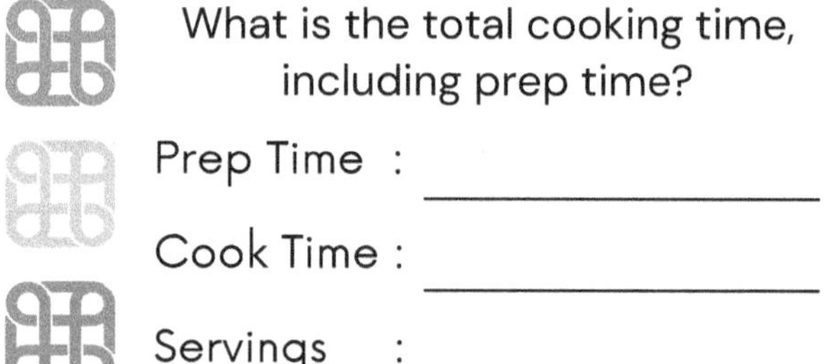

What is the total cooking time, including prep time?

Prep Time : _______________

Cook Time : _______________

Servings   : _______________

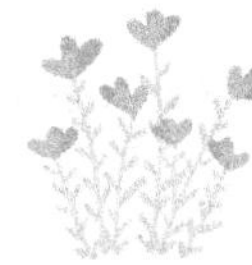

Ingredients:

- 1 cup uncooked quinoa, rinsed
- 1 (15 oz) can black beans, drained and rinsed
- 1 cup diced cucumber
- 1 cup diced tomatoes
- 1/2 cup diced red onion
- 1/2 cup chopped fresh cilantro
- 2 tbsp olive oil
- 2 tbsp lime juice
- 1 tsp ground cumin
- 1/2 tsp chili powder
- 1/4 tsp cayenne pepper (optional, for heat)
- Salt and pepper to taste

1. Cook the quinoa according to package instructions. Allow to cool completely.

2. In a large bowl, combine the cooked quinoa, black beans, cucumber, tomatoes, red onion and cilantro.

3. In a small bowl, whisk together the olive oil, lime juice, cumin, chili powder and cayenne (if using).

4. Pour the dressing over the quinoa salad and toss gently to coat.

5. Season with salt and pepper to taste.

6. Refrigerate the salad for at least 30 minutes to allow the flavors to meld.

7. Serve chilled or at room temperature.

This quinoa and black bean salad is packed with anti-inflammatory ingredients like quinoa, black beans, vegetables, and herbs. The combination of protein, fiber, and healthy fats makes it a nutritious and filling meal. The bright citrus dressing complements the other flavors nicely. This salad is easy to prepare and can be enjoyed by seniors as a light main dish or side.

Is the recipe easy to follow?

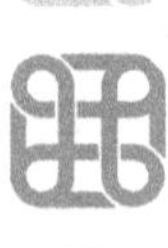
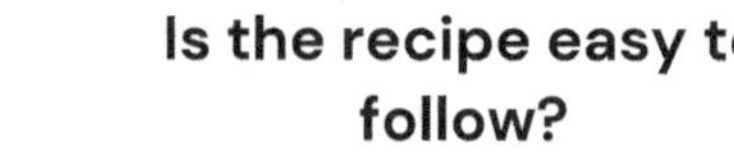

65. Quinoa and Black Bean Salad

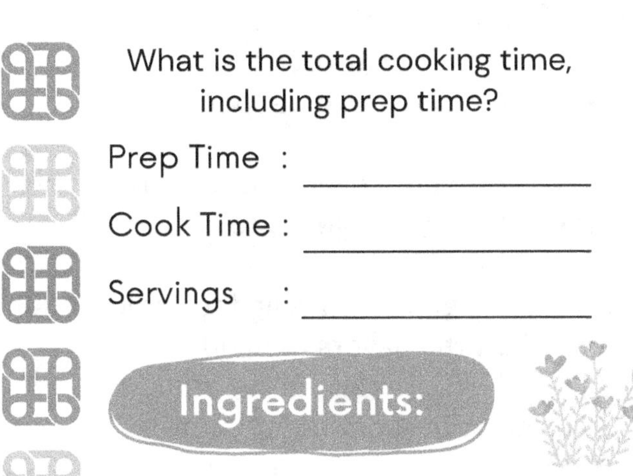

What is the total cooking time, including prep time?

Prep Time : __________________

Cook Time : __________________

Servings   : __________________

Ingredients:

- 4 cups shredded green cabbage
- 1 cup shredded carrots
- 1/4 cup thinly sliced red onion
- 2 tbsp apple cider vinegar
- 1 tbsp olive oil
- 1 tsp Dijon mustard
- 1 tsp honey
- Salt and pepper to taste

Is the recipe easy to follow?

66. Cabbage Slaw with Carrots and Apple Cider Vinegar

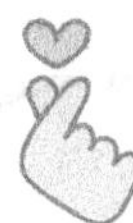

Procedure:

1. In a large bowl, combine the shredded green cabbage, shredded carrots, and thinly sliced red onion.

2. In a small bowl, whisk together the apple cider vinegar, olive oil, Dijon mustard, and honey. Season with salt and pepper.

3. Pour the dressing over the cabbage slaw and toss to coat evenly.

4. Cover and refrigerate the slaw for at least 30 minutes to allow the flavors to meld.

5. Serve the cabbage slaw chilled or at room temperature.

This cabbage slaw is a simple, yet flavorful and nutritious side dish:

- Cabbage is a cruciferous vegetable that is rich in antioxidants and has anti-inflammatory properties.
- Carrots are a good source of beta-carotene, which has anti-inflammatory benefits.
- Apple cider vinegar contains acetic acid, which may help reduce inflammation.
- The Dijon mustard and honey in the dressing provide a nice balance of tanginess and sweetness.

The crunchy texture of the cabbage and carrots, combined with the tangy-sweet dressing, makes this slaw a delightful accompaniment to a variety of meals. It's easy to prepare and can be made in advance, making it a great option for seniors or anyone looking for a healthy, anti-inflammatory side dish.

What are the critical points in the recipe (e.g., temperature control, timing)?

What is the total cooking time, including prep time?

Prep Time : _________________

Cook Time : _________________

Servings   : _________________

Ingredients:

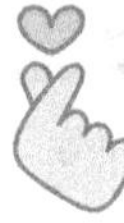

- 1 (15 oz) can chickpeas, drained and rinsed
- 1 cup cherry tomatoes, halved
- 1/2 cup diced cucumber
- 1/4 cup diced red onion
- 2 tbsp chopped fresh parsley
- 2 tbsp olive oil
- 2 tbsp lemon juice
- 1 tsp Dijon mustard
- 1 tsp honey
- 1/2 tsp ground cumin
- Salt and pepper to taste

Is the recipe easy to follow?

67. Chickpea and Tomato Salad

Procedure:

1. In a large bowl, combine the drained and rinsed chickpeas, halved cherry tomatoes, diced cucumber, diced red onion, and chopped parsley.

2. In a small bowl, whisk together the olive oil, lemon juice, Dijon mustard, honey, and ground cumin. Season with salt and pepper.

3. Pour the dressing over the chickpea and tomato mixture and toss gently to coat.

4. Cover and refrigerate the salad for at least 30 minutes to allow the flavors to meld.

5. Serve chilled or at room temperature.

This chickpea and tomato salad is packed with anti-inflammatory ingredients:

- Chickpeas are a good source of plant-based protein, fiber, and complex carbohydrates.
- Tomatoes are rich in the antioxidant lycopene, which has anti-inflammatory properties.
- Cucumber and red onion provide additional vitamins, minerals, and fiber.
- The lemon juice, Dijon mustard, and cumin in the dressing help to reduce inflammation.

The combination of textures and flavors in this salad makes it a delicious and nutritious option for seniors. It's easy to prepare and can be enjoyed as a light main dish or side. The anti-inflammatory ingredients support overall health and may help reduce inflammation.

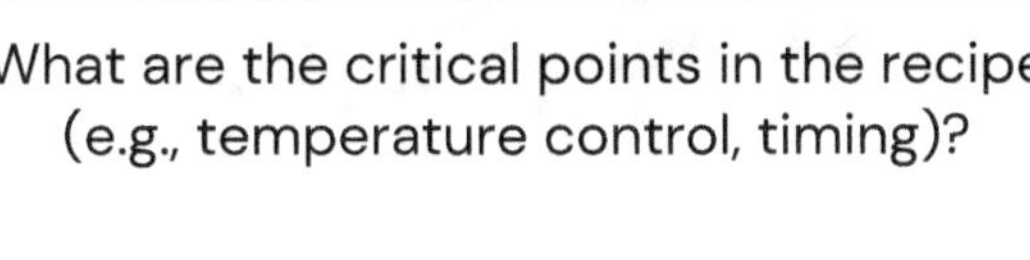

What are the critical points in the recipe (e.g., temperature control, timing)?

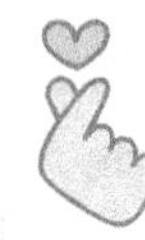

What is the total cooking time, including prep time?

Prep Time : _______________

Cook Time : _______________

Servings : _______________

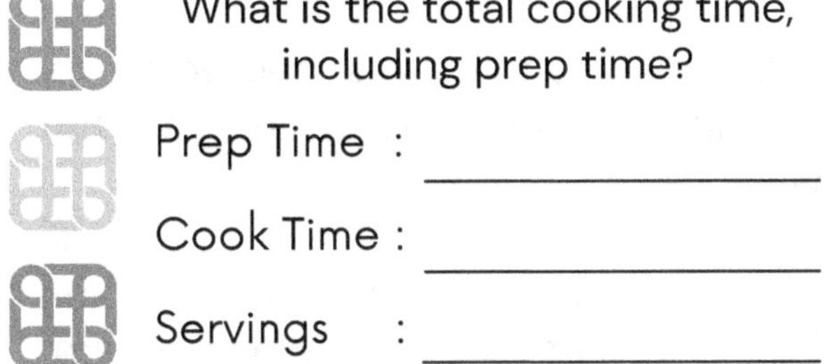

- 4 cups broccoli florets, chopped into bite-size pieces
- 1/2 cup sliced almonds, toasted
- 1/4 cup dried cranberries
- 2 tbsp olive oil
- 2 tbsp apple cider vinegar
- 1 tsp Dijon mustard
- 1 tsp honey
- Salt and pepper to taste

Is the recipe easy to follow?

68. Broccoli and Almond Salad

1. In a large bowl, combine the chopped broccoli florets, toasted almond slices, and dried cranberries.

2. In a small bowl, whisk together the olive oil, apple cider vinegar, Dijon mustard, and honey. Season with salt and pepper.

3. Pour the dressing over the broccoli salad and toss gently to coat.

4. Cover and refrigerate the salad for at least 30 minutes to allow the flavors to meld.

5. Serve chilled or at room temperature.

This broccoli and almond salad is a nutritious and flavorful side dish:

- Broccoli is packed with vitamins, minerals, and antioxidants that have anti-inflammatory properties.
- Almonds provide healthy fats, protein, and fiber.
- Dried cranberries add a touch of sweetness and contain polyphenols with anti-inflammatory benefits.

The crunchy texture of the broccoli and almonds, combined with the chewy cranberries, creates a delightful contrast. The tangy-sweet dressing complements the other flavors nicely.

This salad is easy to prepare and can be made in advance, making it a great option for seniors or anyone looking for a nutritious and flavorful side dish. The combination of anti-inflammatory ingredients makes it a healthy choice.

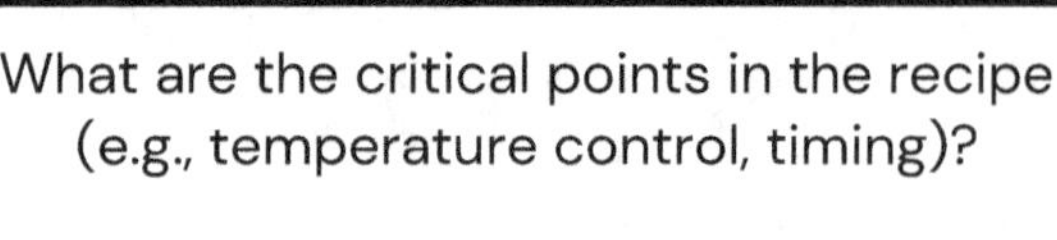 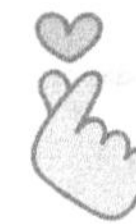

What are the critical points in the recipe (e.g., temperature control, timing)?

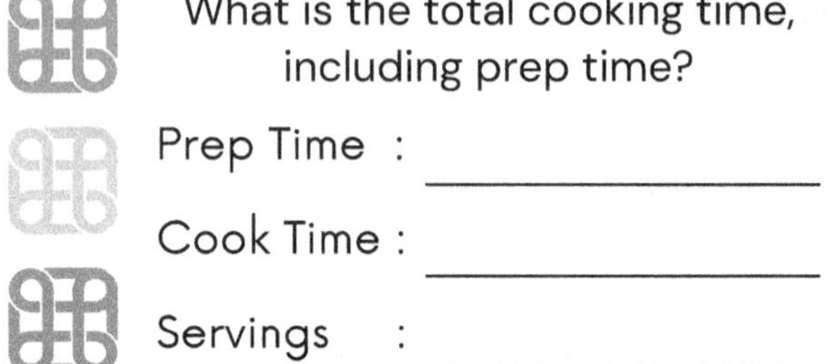

What is the total cooking time, including prep time?

Prep Time : ________________

Cook Time : ________________

Servings : ________________

Ingredients:

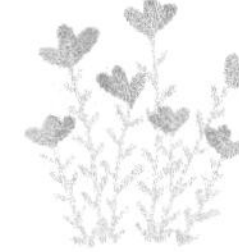

- 3 medium beets, peeled and diced
- 1 cup cooked lentils
- 1/2 cup crumbled feta cheese
- 1/4 cup chopped walnuts, toasted
- 2 tbsp olive oil
- 2 tbsp balsamic vinegar
- 1 tsp Dijon mustard
- 1 tsp honey
- Salt and pepper to taste
- Chopped parsley for garnish (optional)

Is the recipe easy to follow?

69. Roasted Beet and Lentil Salad

1. Preheat your oven to 400°F (200°C).

2. Toss the diced beets with 1 tbsp of the olive oil and season with salt and pepper. Spread the beets on a baking sheet and roast for 20-25 minutes, until tender. Allow to cool slightly.

3. In a large bowl, combine the roasted beets, cooked lentils, crumbled feta cheese, and toasted walnuts.

4. In a small bowl, whisk together the remaining 1 tbsp olive oil, balsamic vinegar, Dijon mustard, and honey. Season with salt and pepper.

5. Drizzle the dressing over the beet and lentil salad and toss gently to coat.

6. Garnish the salad with chopped parsley, if desired.

7. Serve the roasted beet and lentil salad at room temperature or chilled.

This salad is a nutritious and flavorful combination:

- Beets are rich in betalains, which have potent anti-inflammatory properties.
- Lentils provide plant-based protein, fiber, and complex carbohydrates.
- Feta cheese adds a creamy, tangy element, and walnuts provide healthy fats.
- The balsamic vinaigrette ties all the flavors together.

The earthy, sweet beets pair beautifully with the nutty lentils and crunchy walnuts. This salad makes a great light meal or side dish. It's easy to prepare and the combination of nutrients makes it a healthy choice.

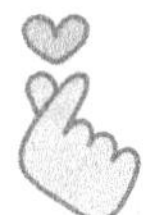

Procedure:

1. In a large bowl, combine the sliced cucumbers, diced avocado, sliced red onion, and chopped cilantro.

2. In a small bowl, whisk together the olive oil, lime juice, honey, and ground cumin. Season with salt and pepper.

3. Pour the dressing over the cucumber and avocado salad and toss gently to coat.

4. Refrigerate the salad for at least 15 minutes to allow the flavors to meld.

5. Serve chilled or at room temperature.

This cucumber and avocado salad is packed with anti-inflammatory ingredients:

- Cucumbers are hydrating and contain antioxidants that can help reduce inflammation.
- Avocados are rich in healthy monounsaturated fats, which have anti-inflammatory properties.
- Cilantro contains compounds that may help reduce inflammation.
- Lime juice and olive oil also have anti-inflammatory benefits.

The combination of crunchy cucumbers, creamy avocado, and the bright, tangy dressing creates a refreshing and flavorful salad. It's an easy-to-prepare dish that can be enjoyed as a light main or side for seniors.

The anti-inflammatory nutrients in this salad make it a great choice for supporting overall health and potentially reducing inflammation in the body.

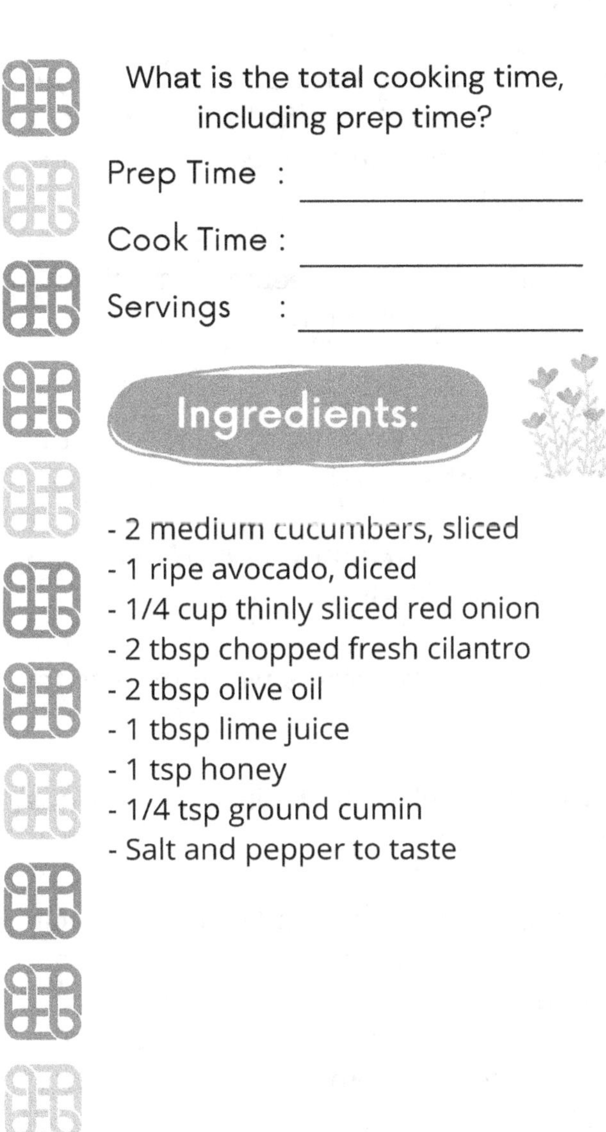

What is the total cooking time, including prep time?

Prep Time : _______________

Cook Time : _______________

Servings   : _______________

Ingredients:

- 2 medium cucumbers, sliced
- 1 ripe avocado, diced
- 1/4 cup thinly sliced red onion
- 2 tbsp chopped fresh cilantro
- 2 tbsp olive oil
- 1 tbsp lime juice
- 1 tsp honey
- 1/4 tsp ground cumin
- Salt and pepper to taste

Is the recipe easy to follow?

70. *Cucumber and Avocado Salad*

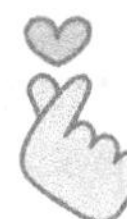

What is the total cooking time, including prep time?

Prep Time : _________________

Cook Time : _________________

Servings : _________________

Ingredients:

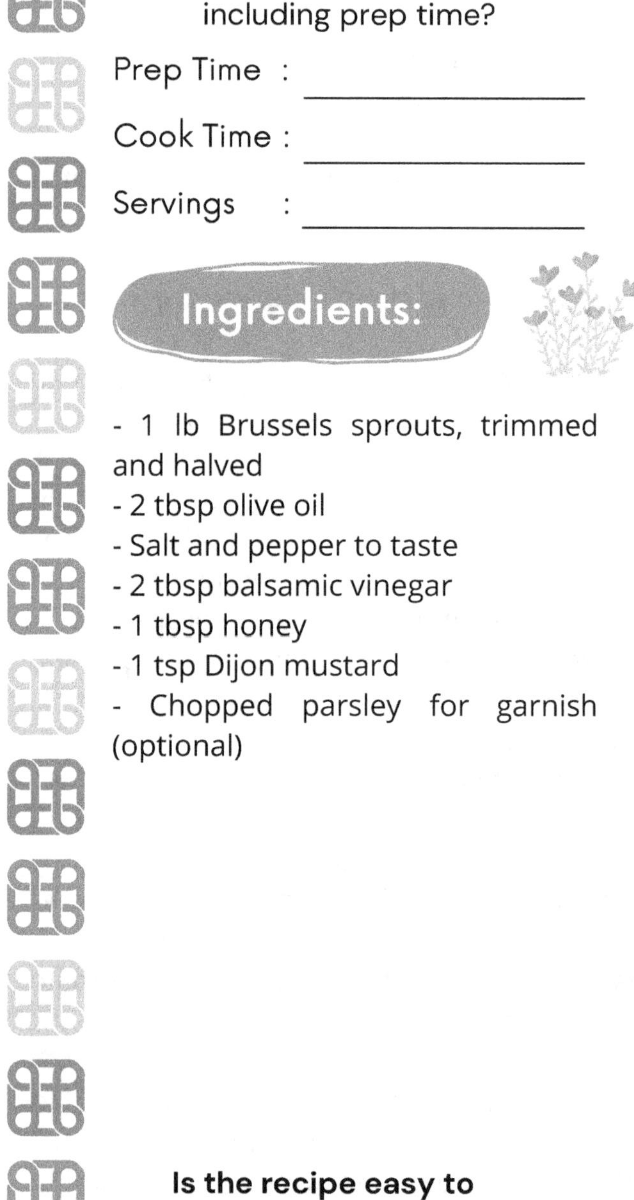

- 1 lb Brussels sprouts, trimmed and halved
- 2 tbsp olive oil
- Salt and pepper to taste
- 2 tbsp balsamic vinegar
- 1 tbsp honey
- 1 tsp Dijon mustard
- Chopped parsley for garnish (optional)

Is the recipe easy to follow?

🙂   🙁

71. Roasted Brussels Sprouts with Balsamic Glaze

1. Preheat your oven to 400°F (200°C).

2. In a large bowl, toss the trimmed and halved Brussels sprouts with the olive oil. Season with salt and pepper.

3. Spread the Brussels sprouts in a single layer on a baking sheet. Roast for 20-25 minutes, tossing halfway, until the sprouts are tender and lightly browned.

4. In a small bowl, whisk together the balsamic vinegar, honey, and Dijon mustard.

5. Transfer the roasted Brussels sprouts to a serving bowl. Drizzle the balsamic glaze over the top and toss gently to coat.

6. Garnish the roasted Brussels sprouts with chopped parsley, if desired.

7. Serve the Brussels sprouts warm or at room temperature.

This roasted Brussels sprouts dish is a delicious and nutritious side:

- Brussels sprouts are a cruciferous vegetable rich in antioxidants and anti-inflammatory compounds.
- The balsamic vinegar and honey create a sweet-tart glaze that complements the natural flavors of the Brussels sprouts.
- Roasting the Brussels sprouts brings out their natural sweetness and gives them a delightful texture.

This recipe is suitable for seniors and anyone looking to incorporate more anti-inflammatory foods into their diet.

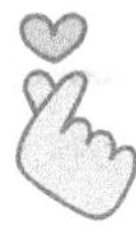

What are the critical points in the recipe (e.g., temperature control, timing)?

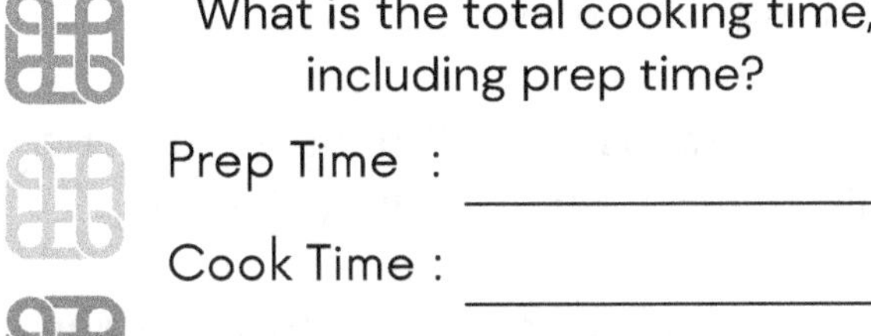

What is the total cooking time, including prep time?

Prep Time : _________________

Cook Time : _________________

Servings : _________________

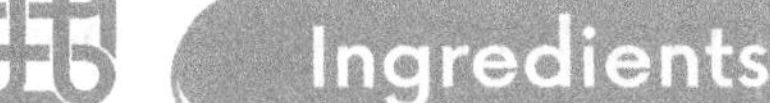 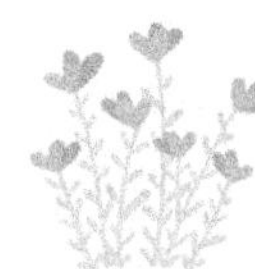

Ingredients:

- 1 lb broccoli florets
- 2 tbsp olive oil
- 2 tbsp fresh lemon juice
- 1 tsp lemon zest
- 1/4 tsp garlic powder
- Salt and pepper to taste
- Chopped parsley for garnish (optional)

Is the recipe easy to follow?

72. Steamed Broccoli with Lemon

1. Fill a large pot with about 1 inch of water and bring to a boil. Place a steamer basket in the pot.

2. Add the broccoli florets to the steamer basket, cover, and steam for 5-7 minutes, until the broccoli is tender but still crisp.

3. Carefully transfer the steamed broccoli to a serving bowl.

4. In a small bowl, whisk together the olive oil, lemon juice, lemon zest, and garlic powder.

5. Drizzle the lemon dressing over the hot broccoli and toss gently to coat.

6. Season the broccoli with salt and pepper to taste.

7. Garnish with chopped parsley, if desired.

8. Serve the steamed broccoli warm or at room temperature.

This simple steamed broccoli dish is packed with anti-inflammatory benefits:

- Broccoli is a cruciferous vegetable rich in antioxidants and anti-inflammatory compounds.
- Lemon juice and zest provide vitamin C, which has potent anti-inflammatory properties.
- Olive oil contains healthy monounsaturated fats that can help reduce inflammation.

The bright, lemony flavor complements the natural sweetness of the broccoli. This easy-to-prepare side dish is perfect for seniors looking to incorporate more anti-inflammatory foods into their diet. It's a nutritious and flavorful way to enjoy broccoli.

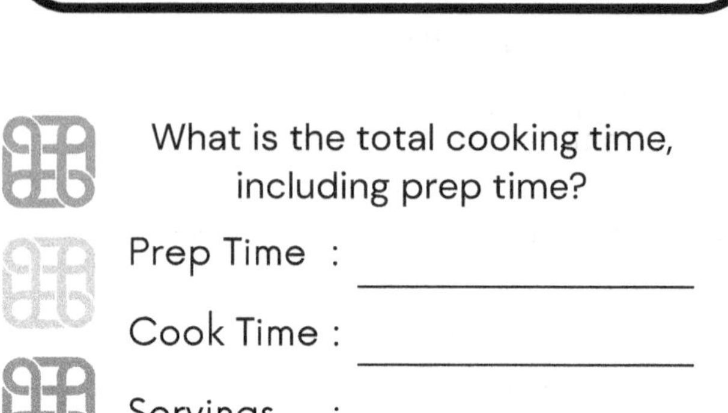

What is the total cooking time, including prep time?

Prep Time : _______________

Cook Time : _______________

Servings   : _______________

Ingredients:

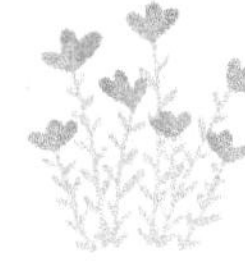

- 1 lb asparagus, woody ends trimmed
- 2 tbsp olive oil
- 3 cloves garlic, minced
- 1/2 tsp lemon zest
- 1/4 tsp crushed red pepper flakes (optional)
- Salt and pepper to taste
- Lemon wedges for serving

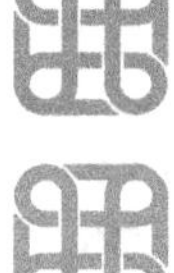
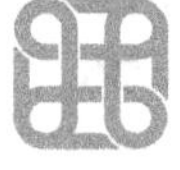
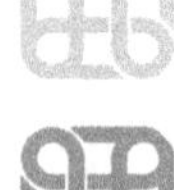
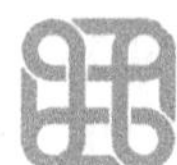

Is the recipe easy to follow?

73. Grilled Asparagus with Garlic

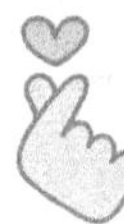

Procedure:

1. Preheat your grill or grill pan to medium-high heat.

2. In a large bowl, toss the trimmed asparagus spears with the olive oil, minced garlic, lemon zest, and crushed red pepper flakes (if using). Season with salt and pepper.

3. Grill the asparagus for 5-7 minutes, turning occasionally, until tender and lightly charred.

4. Transfer the grilled asparagus to a serving platter.

5. Serve the asparagus warm, with lemon wedges on the side.

This grilled asparagus dish is an excellent choice for seniors looking to incorporate anti-inflammatory foods into their diet:

- Asparagus is a nutrient-dense vegetable that is rich in antioxidants and anti-inflammatory compounds.
- Garlic contains sulfur compounds that have potent anti-inflammatory properties.
- Lemon zest adds a bright, refreshing note and provides vitamin C, which has anti-inflammatory benefits.
- Olive oil is a source of healthy monounsaturated fats that can help reduce inflammation.

The simplicity of this recipe allows the natural flavors of the asparagus to shine, while the garlic, lemon, and optional red pepper flakes add a flavorful twist. Grilling the asparagus gives it a delicious smoky flavor and tender-crisp texture.

What are the critical points in the recipe (e.g., temperature control, timing)?

What is the total cooking time, including prep time?

Prep Time : ________________

Cook Time : ________________

Servings   : ________________

- 1 large head of cauliflower, cut into florets
- 2 tbsp olive oil
- 2 tbsp unsweetened almond milk (or regular milk)
- 2 tbsp chopped fresh chives
- 1 tsp garlic powder
- 1/2 tsp ground black pepper
- 1/4 tsp salt

Is the recipe easy to follow?

74. Mashed Cauliflower with Chives

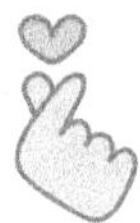

1. In a large pot, bring a few inches of water to a boil. Add the cauliflower florets, cover, and steam for 10-12 minutes, until very tender.

2. Drain the cauliflower and transfer it to a food processor or high-powered blender.

3. Add the olive oil, almond milk, chopped chives, garlic powder, black pepper, and salt. Blend or process until smooth and creamy, scraping down the sides as needed.

4. Taste and adjust seasoning as desired.

5. Transfer the mashed cauliflower to a serving bowl.

6. Serve the mashed cauliflower warm, garnished with additional chopped chives if desired.

This mashed cauliflower dish is an excellent anti-inflammatory option for seniors:

- Cauliflower is a cruciferous vegetable rich in antioxidants and anti-inflammatory compounds.
- Olive oil provides healthy monounsaturated fats that can help reduce inflammation.
- Chives contain sulfur compounds with anti-inflammatory properties.
- The simple seasoning with garlic powder, black pepper, and a touch of salt enhances the natural flavors.

The creamy, smooth texture of the mashed cauliflower makes it a comforting and easy-to-digest side dish. It can be enjoyed on its own or paired with other anti-inflammatory main dishes.

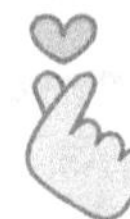

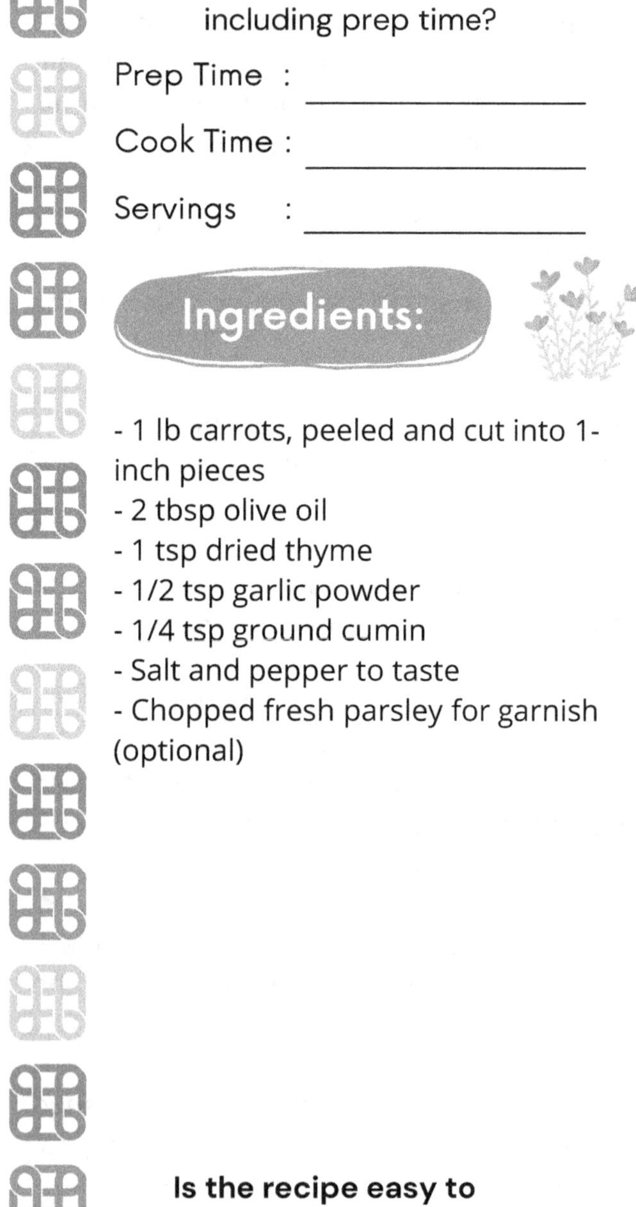

What is the total cooking time, including prep time?

Prep Time : _______________

Cook Time : _______________

Servings   : _______________

Ingredients:

- 1 lb carrots, peeled and cut into 1-inch pieces
- 2 tbsp olive oil
- 1 tsp dried thyme
- 1/2 tsp garlic powder
- 1/4 tsp ground cumin
- Salt and pepper to taste
- Chopped fresh parsley for garnish (optional)

Is the recipe easy to follow?

75. Roasted Carrots with Thyme

1. Preheat your oven to 400°F (200°C).

2. In a large bowl, toss the peeled and cut carrots with the olive oil, dried thyme, garlic powder, and ground cumin. Season with salt and pepper.

3. Spread the seasoned carrots in a single layer on a baking sheet.

4. Roast the carrots for 20-25 minutes, tossing halfway, until they are tender and lightly browned.

5. Transfer the roasted carrots to a serving dish.

6. Garnish the carrots with chopped fresh parsley, if desired.

7. Serve the roasted carrots warm.

This roasted carrot dish is an excellent anti-inflammatory option for seniors:

- Carrots are rich in beta-carotene, an antioxidant with anti-inflammatory properties.
- Thyme contains thymol, a compound with potent anti-inflammatory effects.
- Garlic powder and cumin also have anti-inflammatory benefits.
- Olive oil provides healthy monounsaturated fats that can help reduce inflammation.

The combination of sweet, earthy carrots and the aromatic herbs and spices creates a delicious and nutritious side dish. Roasting the carrots brings out their natural sweetness and gives them a tender, caramelized texture.

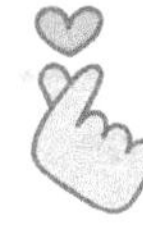

What is the total cooking time, including prep time?

Prep Time : _______________

Cook Time : _______________

Servings   : _______________

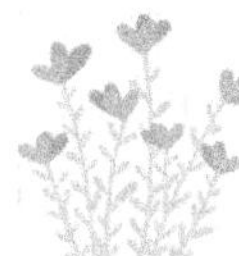

Ingredients:

- 1 cup uncooked quinoa, rinsed
- 2 cups low-sodium vegetable or chicken broth
- 2 tbsp olive oil
- 1 onion, diced
- 3 cloves garlic, minced
- 1 cup diced zucchini
- 1/2 cup diced bell pepper
- 1/4 cup chopped fresh parsley
- 2 tbsp chopped fresh basil
- 1 tsp dried oregano
- Salt and pepper to taste

1. In a medium saucepan, combine the rinsed quinoa and broth. Bring to a boil, then reduce heat, cover, and simmer for 15-20 minutes, until the quinoa is tender and the liquid is absorbed.

2. In a large skillet, heat the olive oil over medium heat. Add the diced onion and sauté for 5 minutes until translucent.

3. Add the minced garlic, diced zucchini, and diced bell pepper to the skillet. Cook for an additional 5-7 minutes, stirring occasionally, until the vegetables are tender.

4. Fluff the cooked quinoa with a fork and add it to the skillet with the sautéed vegetables.

5. Stir in the chopped parsley, basil, and dried oregano. Season with salt and pepper to taste.

6. Cook for 2-3 minutes, stirring frequently, to allow the flavors to meld.

7. Serve the quinoa pilaf warm, garnished with additional fresh herbs if desired.

This quinoa pilaf is packed with anti-inflammatory ingredients:

- Quinoa is a nutrient-dense grain that provides protein, fiber, and complex carbohydrates.
- Zucchini, bell peppers, and herbs like parsley and basil are rich in antioxidants and have anti-inflammatory properties.

The combination of textures and flavors in this dish makes it a delicious and nutritious option for seniors. It's easy to prepare and can be enjoyed as a main course or a side. The anti-inflammatory nutrients support overall health and may help reduce inflammation in the body.

Is the recipe easy to follow?

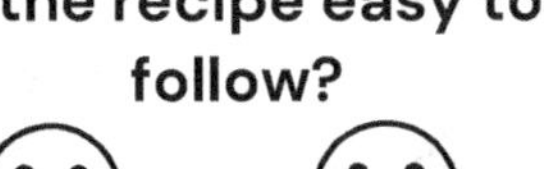

76. Quinoa Pilaf with Herbs

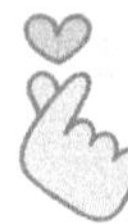

Procedure:

What is the total cooking time,
including prep time?

Prep Time : _______________

Cook Time : _______________

Servings   : _______________

Ingredients:

- 1 lb fresh spinach, washed and stems removed
- 2 tbsp olive oil
- 3 cloves garlic, minced
- 1/4 tsp red pepper flakes (optional)
- Salt and pepper to taste

Is the recipe easy to follow?

77. Sautéed Spinach with Garlic

1. In a large skillet or sauté pan, heat the olive oil over medium heat.

2. Add the minced garlic and red pepper flakes (if using) to the pan. Cook for 1-2 minutes, stirring frequently, until the garlic is fragrant and lightly golden.

3. Add the fresh spinach to the pan in batches, stirring constantly, until the spinach is wilted down and reduced in volume, about 3-5 minutes total.

4. Season the sautéed spinach with salt and pepper to taste. Serve the sautéed spinach warm, as a side dish.

This simple sautéed spinach dish is a nutritious and flavorful option:

- Spinach is an excellent source of vitamins, minerals, and antioxidants that have anti-inflammatory properties.
- Garlic contains sulfur compounds that also have anti-inflammatory benefits.
- The red pepper flakes (optional) can provide a subtle heat and additional antioxidants.
- Olive oil is a healthy fat that can help reduce inflammation.

The quick sauté method preserves the nutrients in the spinach while infusing it with the aromatic garlic flavor. This dish is easy to prepare and can be enjoyed as a side or incorporated into other meals.

Sautéed spinach with garlic is a great way for seniors to increase their intake of anti-inflammatory foods. It's a simple, versatile recipe that can be adjusted to personal taste preferences.

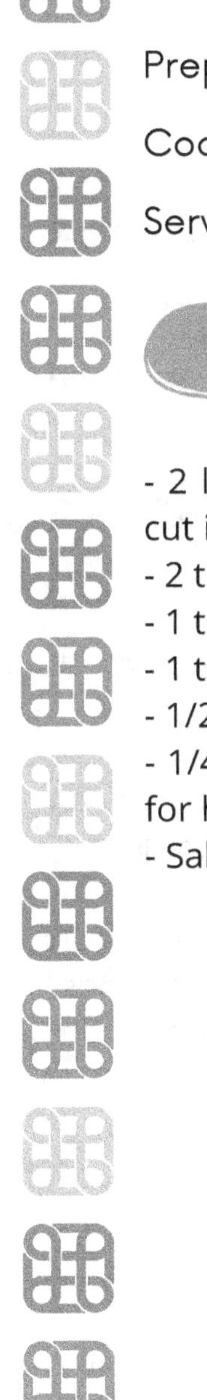

What is the total cooking time, including prep time?

Prep Time : _______________

Cook Time : _______________

Servings   : _______________

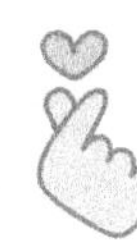

Ingredients:

- 2 lbs sweet potatoes, peeled and cut into 1/2-inch thick fry shapes
- 2 tbsp olive oil
- 1 tsp ground cumin
- 1 tsp paprika
- 1/2 tsp garlic powder
- 1/4 tsp cayenne pepper (optional, for heat)
- Salt and pepper to taste

Is the recipe easy to follow?

78. Sweet Potato Fries

Procedure:

1. Preheat your oven to 400°F (200°C). Line a large baking sheet with parchment paper.

2. In a large bowl, toss the cut sweet potato fries with the olive oil, cumin, paprika, garlic powder, and cayenne pepper (if using). Season with salt and pepper.

3. Spread the seasoned sweet potato fries in a single layer on the prepared baking sheet.

4. Bake for 20-25 minutes, flipping the fries halfway, until they are tender and lightly browned.

5. Remove the sweet potato fries from the oven and serve hot.

These sweet potato fries are an anti-inflammatory option for seniors:

- Sweet potatoes are rich in beta-carotene, an antioxidant with anti-inflammatory properties.
- Cumin, paprika, and garlic powder provide additional anti-inflammatory benefits.

- Cayenne pepper (optional) contains capsaicin, which has been shown to have anti-inflammatory effects.

The combination of spices and roasting method brings out the natural sweetness of the sweet potatoes while creating a crispy exterior. This makes for a delicious and nutritious side dish or snack.

Seniors can enjoy these sweet potato fries as a healthier alternative to traditional french fries. The anti-inflammatory ingredients support overall health and may help reduce inflammation in the body.

What is the total cooking time, including prep time?

Prep Time : ___________________

Cook Time : ___________________

Servings : ___________________

Ingredients:

- 1 head of cauliflower, cut into florets
- 2 tbsp olive oil
- 1 tsp ground turmeric
- 1/2 tsp ground cumin
- 1/4 tsp ground coriander
- 1/4 tsp garlic powder
- Salt and pepper to taste
- Chopped fresh parsley for garnish (optional)

Is the recipe easy to follow?

☺   ☹

79. Cauliflower Rice with Turmeric

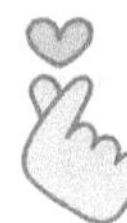

Procedure:

1. In a food processor, pulse the cauliflower florets in batches until they are broken down into small, rice-like pieces.

2. In a large skillet, heat the olive oil over medium heat.

3. Add the riced cauliflower, turmeric, cumin, coriander, and garlic powder to the skillet. Stir to combine.

4. Cook the cauliflower rice, stirring occasionally, for 5-7 minutes, until it is tender and the spices are fragrant.

5. Season the cauliflower rice with salt and pepper to taste.

6. Transfer the turmeric cauliflower rice to a serving bowl.

7. Garnish with chopped fresh parsley, if desired. Serve the cauliflower rice warm.

This turmeric-infused cauliflower rice dish is an excellent anti-inflammatory option for seniors:

- Cauliflower is a cruciferous vegetable rich in antioxidants and anti-inflammatory compounds.
- Turmeric contains curcumin, a powerful anti-inflammatory compound.
- Cumin and coriander also have anti-inflammatory properties.
- Olive oil provides healthy monounsaturated fats that can help reduce inflammation.

The vibrant yellow color and earthy, aromatic flavors of this cauliflower rice make it a delicious and nutritious side dish. It's easy to prepare and can be enjoyed on its own or as a base for other anti-inflammatory meals.

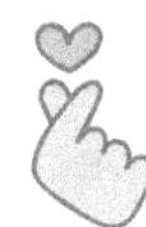

What are the critical points in the recipe (e.g., temperature control, timing)?

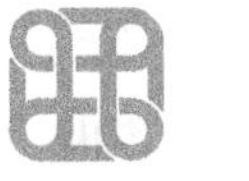

What is the total cooking time, including prep time?

Prep Time : _______________

Cook Time : _______________

Servings   : _______________

Ingredients:

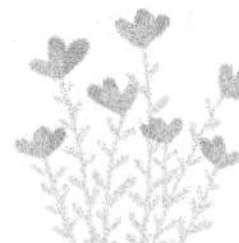

- 2 medium zucchini, sliced lengthwise into 1/2-inch thick strips
- 2 medium yellow squash, sliced lengthwise into 1/2-inch thick strips
- 2 tbsp olive oil
- 1 tsp dried oregano
- 1 tsp dried basil
- 1/2 tsp garlic powder
- Salt and pepper to taste
- Lemon wedges for serving

Is the recipe easy to follow?

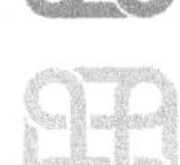 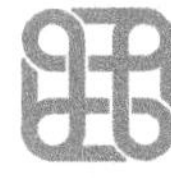 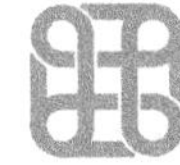  

80. Grilled Zucchini and Squash

1. Preheat your grill or grill pan to medium-high heat.

2. In a large bowl, toss the zucchini and squash strips with the olive oil, oregano, basil, garlic powder, salt, and pepper until evenly coated.

3. Grill the zucchini and squash slices for 3-4 minutes per side, or until they are tender and have nice grill marks.

4. Transfer the grilled vegetables to a serving platter.

5. Serve the grilled zucchini and squash warm, with lemon wedges on the side.

This grilled vegetable dish is an excellent choice for seniors looking to incorporate anti-inflammatory foods into their diet:

- Zucchini and squash are low in calories and high in fiber, vitamins, and antioxidants that can help reduce inflammation.
- The herbs and spices used in the seasoning, such as oregano and basil, also have anti-inflammatory properties.
- Grilling the vegetables brings out their natural sweetness and adds a delicious smoky flavor.

The simplicity of this recipe allows the natural flavors of the vegetables to shine. Seniors can enjoy this dish as a side or a light main course. The combination of nutrients and anti-inflammatory components makes it a healthy and satisfying option.

Remember to adjust the cooking time as needed, as seniors may prefer their vegetables to be more tender. Serve with lemon wedges to add a bright, refreshing note.

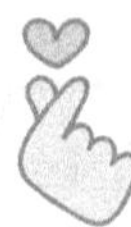

What is the total cooking time,
including prep time?

Prep Time : ___________________

Cook Time : ___________________

Servings   : ___________________

Ingredients:

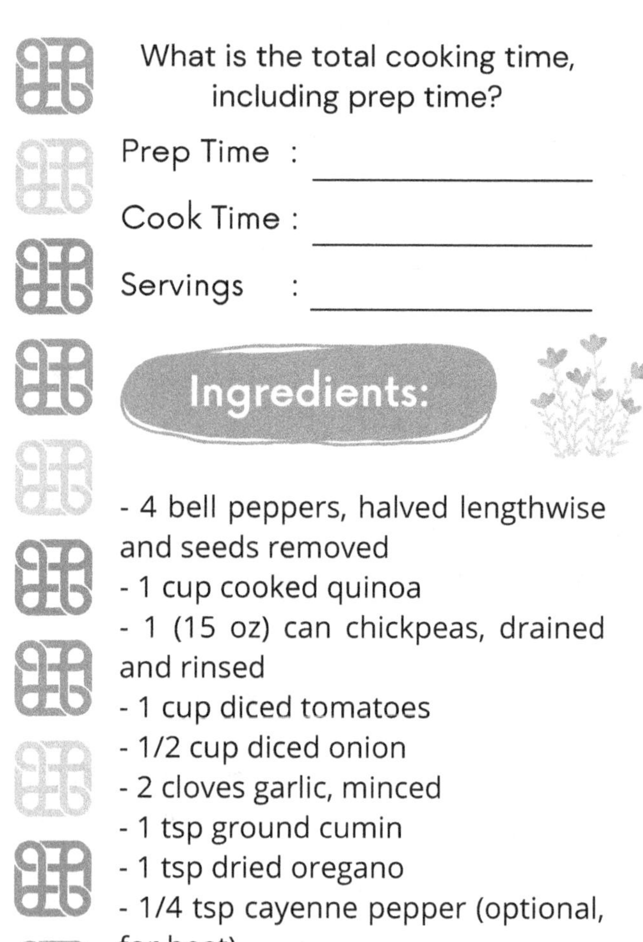

- 4 bell peppers, halved lengthwise and seeds removed
- 1 cup cooked quinoa
- 1 (15 oz) can chickpeas, drained and rinsed
- 1 cup diced tomatoes
- 1/2 cup diced onion
- 2 cloves garlic, minced
- 1 tsp ground cumin
- 1 tsp dried oregano
- 1/4 tsp cayenne pepper (optional, for heat)
- Salt and pepper to taste
- 1/2 cup crumbled feta cheese (optional)
- Chopped fresh parsley for garnish

Is the recipe easy to follow?

81. *Stuffed Bell Peppers with Quinoa and Chickpeas*

1. Preheat your oven to 375°F (190°C).

2. Arrange the bell pepper halves in a baking dish or on a rimmed baking sheet.

3. In a large bowl, combine the cooked quinoa, chickpeas, diced tomatoes, onion, garlic, cumin, oregano, and cayenne (if using). Season with salt and pepper.

4. Spoon the quinoa and chickpea mixture evenly into the bell pepper halves.

5. If using, sprinkle the crumbled feta cheese over the top of the stuffed peppers.

6. Bake the stuffed peppers for 25-30 minutes, until the peppers are tender and the filling is heated through.

7. Remove the stuffed peppers from the oven and garnish with chopped fresh parsley.

8. Serve the stuffed bell peppers warm.

This dish is packed with anti-inflammatory ingredients:

- Bell peppers are rich in vitamins and antioxidants that have anti-inflammatory properties.
- Quinoa is a nutrient-dense grain that provides protein, fiber, and complex carbohydrates.
- Chickpeas are a good source of plant-based protein and fiber.
- Cumin, oregano, and garlic have anti-inflammatory benefits.
- Feta cheese (optional) provides calcium and probiotics that may help reduce inflammation.

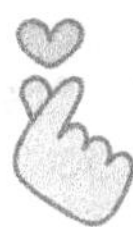

What is the total cooking time, including prep time?

Prep Time : ________________

Cook Time : ________________

Servings   : ________________

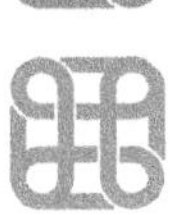
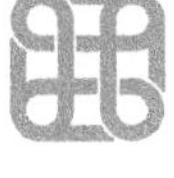

Ingredients:

- 1 medium spaghetti squash, halved lengthwise and seeds removed
- 2 tbsp olive oil
- Salt and pepper to taste
- 1 (24 oz) jar marinara sauce
- Grated Parmesan cheese (optional)
- Chopped fresh basil (optional)

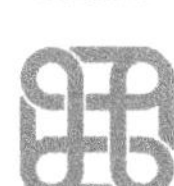
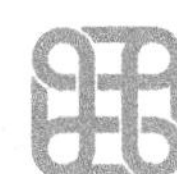

Is the recipe easy to follow?

82. Spaghetti Squash with Marinara Sauce

1. Preheat your oven to 400°F (200°C).

2. Place the spaghetti squash halves cut-side up on a baking sheet. Drizzle the squash with 1 tbsp of the olive oil and season with salt and pepper.

3. Roast the spaghetti squash for 40-50 minutes, until tender when pierced with a fork.

4. Remove the spaghetti squash from the oven and let it cool slightly.

5. Using a fork, gently scrape the flesh of the spaghetti squash to create long, spaghetti-like strands.

6. In a large skillet, heat the remaining 1 tbsp of olive oil over medium heat. Add the spaghetti squash strands and sauté for 2-3 minutes to heat through.

7. Pour the marinara sauce over the spaghetti squash and toss to combine.

8. Serve the spaghetti squash with marinara sauce, topped with grated Parmesan cheese and chopped fresh basil, if desired.

This spaghetti squash dish is a healthy and flavorful alternative to traditional pasta:

- Spaghetti squash is a low-calorie, nutrient-dense vegetable that is high in fiber and vitamins.
- Marinara sauce is a good source of lycopene, an antioxidant with anti-inflammatory properties.
- Olive oil provides healthy monounsaturated fats that can help reduce inflammation.

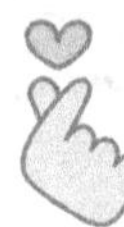

What are the critical points in the recipe (e.g., temperature control, timing)?

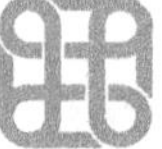

What is the total cooking time, including prep time?

Prep Time : _______________

Cook Time : _______________

Servings : _______________

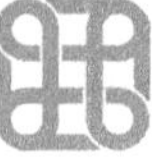 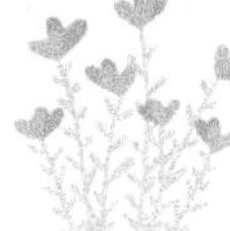

Ingredients:

- 1 block of extra-firm tofu, pressed and cubed
- 2 tbsp vegetable oil
- 1 red bell pepper, sliced
- 1 cup broccoli florets
- 1 cup sliced mushrooms
- 1 cup snow peas or snap peas
- 3 cloves garlic, minced
- 1 tbsp grated ginger
- 2 tbsp low-sodium soy sauce or tamari
- 1 tbsp rice vinegar
- 1 tsp sesame oil
- Salt and pepper to taste
- Cooked rice or noodles, for serving

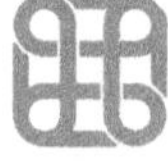

Is the recipe easy to follow?

83. Vegan Tofu Stir-Fry with Vegetables

1. Press the tofu for 30 minutes to remove excess moisture. Cut into 1-inch cubes.

2. Heat the vegetable oil in a large skillet or wok over medium-high heat. Add the tofu cubes and cook for 3-4 minutes per side until lightly browned. Remove tofu from the pan and set aside.

3. Add the bell pepper, broccoli, mushrooms, and snow peas to the pan. Stir-fry for 3-4 minutes until vegetables are tender-crisp.

4. Add the garlic and ginger and cook for 1 minute until fragrant.

5. Return the tofu to the pan. Pour in the soy sauce, rice vinegar, and sesame oil. Toss everything together and cook for 2-3 minutes until heated through.

6. Season with salt and pepper to taste.

7. Serve the tofu stir-fry immediately over cooked rice or noodles.

Enjoy your delicious and healthy vegan tofu stir-fry!

What is the total cooking time,
including prep time?

Prep Time : _______________

Cook Time : _______________

Servings   : _______________

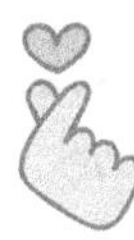

Ingredients:

Meatballs:
- 1 cup cooked brown rice
- 1 (15 oz) can chickpeas, drained and rinsed
- 1 cup rolled oats
- 1/2 cup finely chopped onion
- 3 cloves garlic, minced
- 1 tsp dried oregano
- 1 tsp dried basil
- 1/2 tsp ground cumin
- 1/4 tsp cayenne pepper
- Salt and pepper to taste

Tomato Sauce:
- 1 tbsp olive oil
- 1 onion, diced
- 3 cloves garlic, minced
- 1 (28 oz) can diced tomatoes
- 2 tbsp tomato paste
- 1 tsp dried oregano
- 1 tsp dried basil
- Salt and pepper to taste

84. Vegan Meatballs with Tomato Sauce

Procedure:

For the Meatballs:
1. In a food processor, combine the cooked rice, chickpeas, oats, onion, garlic, oregano, basil, cumin, and cayenne. Pulse until well combined but still slightly chunky.
2. Form the mixture into 1-inch meatballs and place on a parchment-lined baking sheet.
3. Bake at 375°F for 20-25 minutes, flipping halfway, until lightly browned.

For the Tomato Sauce:
1. In a saucepan, heat the olive oil over medium heat. Add the onion and garlic and sauté for 3-4 minutes until translucent.
2. Stir in the diced tomatoes, tomato paste, oregano, and basil. Season with salt and pepper.
3. Simmer the sauce for 10-15 minutes, stirring occasionally, until thickened.

To Serve:
1. Add the baked meatballs to the tomato sauce and gently toss to coat.
2. Serve the vegan meatballs and sauce over whole grain pasta, zucchini noodles, or on their own.

The key anti-inflammatory ingredients in this recipe include:
- Chickpeas - high in fiber, protein, and anti-inflammatory nutrients
- Olive oil - rich in anti-inflammatory monounsaturated fats
- Herbs like oregano and basil - contain antioxidants and anti-inflammatory compounds
- Spices like cumin and cayenne - have potent anti-inflammatory properties

This makes it a great option for seniors looking to incorporate more anti-inflammatory foods into their diet.

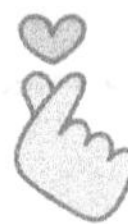

Procedure:

1. In a large pot or Dutch oven, heat the olive oil over medium heat. Add the diced onion and sauté for 5 minutes until translucent.

2. Add the minced garlic, cumin, coriander, paprika, ginger, and cayenne (if using). Cook for 1 minute, stirring constantly, until fragrant.

3. Stir in the drained and rinsed chickpeas, diced tomatoes, butternut squash, zucchini, bell pepper, and vegetable broth. Season with salt and pepper.

4. Bring the tagine to a simmer, then reduce heat and let it cook for 20-25 minutes, until the vegetables are tender.

5. Taste and adjust seasonings as needed.

6. Serve the chickpea and vegetable tagine hot, garnished with chopped cilantro.

This tagine is packed with anti-inflammatory ingredients:

- Chickpeas provide plant-based protein, fiber, and complex carbohydrates.
- Butternut squash, zucchini, and bell peppers are rich in antioxidants and anti-inflammatory vitamins.
- The spices, including cumin, coriander, and ginger, have potent anti-inflammatory properties.
- Olive oil contains healthy monounsaturated fats that can help reduce inflammation.

The combination of aromatic spices, tender vegetables, and hearty chickpeas creates a flavorful and nourishing stew-like dish. It's easy to prepare and can be enjoyed as a main course or side by seniors.

What is the total cooking time, including prep time?

Prep Time : _______________

Cook Time : _______________

Servings : _______________

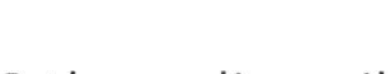

Ingredients:

- 2 tbsp olive oil
- 1 onion, diced
- 3 cloves garlic, minced
- 1 tsp ground cumin
- 1 tsp ground coriander
- 1 tsp paprika
- 1/2 tsp ground ginger
- 1/4 tsp cayenne pepper (optional, for heat)
- 1 (15 oz) can chickpeas, drained and rinsed
- 1 (14 oz) can diced tomatoes
- 2 cups diced butternut squash
- 1 cup diced zucchini
- 1 cup diced bell pepper
- 1 cup low-sodium vegetable broth
- Salt and pepper to taste
- Chopped cilantro for garnish

Is the recipe easy to follow?

85. Chickpea and Vegetable Tagine

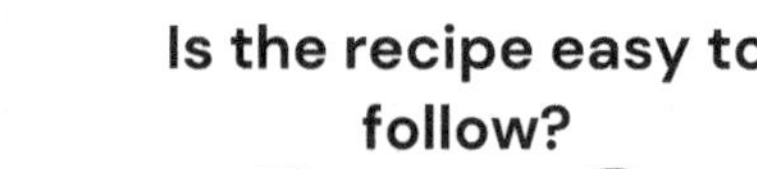

Procedure:

1. Preheat oven to 375°F.

For the Filling:
1. In a medium saucepan, combine the lentils and vegetable broth. Bring to a boil, then reduce heat and simmer for 20-25 minutes until lentils are tender. Drain any excess liquid and set aside.
2. In a large skillet, heat the olive oil over medium heat. Add the onion and sauté for 5 minutes until translucent.
3. Add the mushrooms and garlic and cook for 3-4 minutes until mushrooms are softened.
4. Stir in the thyme, rosemary, tomato paste, and flour. Cook for 1 minute.
5. Gradually whisk in the almond milk and cook for 2-3 minutes until thickened.
6. Add the cooked lentils and season with salt and pepper.

For the Mashed Potato Topping:
1. Place the potato chunks in a large pot and cover with water. Bring to a boil and cook for 15-20 minutes until very tender. Drain.
2. In a large bowl, mash the potatoes with the almond milk and vegan butter until smooth and creamy. Season with salt.

Assemble and Bake:
1. Spread the lentil mushroom filling into a 9x13 inch baking dish.
2. Spoon the mashed potatoes over top and spread evenly.
3. Bake for 30-35 minutes until the potatoes are lightly browned on top.
4. Let stand for 5-10 minutes before serving.

Enjoy this hearty and comforting vegan shepherd's pie!

What is the total cooking time,
including prep time?

Prep Time : _______________

Cook Time : _______________

Servings   : _______________

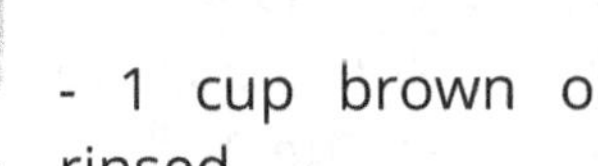

Ingredients:

- 1 cup brown or green lentils, rinsed
- 4 cups vegetable broth
- 1 tbsp olive oil
- 1 onion, diced
- 8 oz mushrooms, sliced
- 3 cloves garlic, minced
- 2 tsp dried thyme
- 1 tsp dried rosemary
- 2 tbsp tomato paste
- 2 tbsp all-purpose flour
- 1 cup unsweetened almond milk
- Salt and pepper to taste

Mashed Potato Topping:
- 3 lbs Yukon Gold potatoes, peeled and cut into 1-inch chunks
- 1/2 cup unsweetened almond milk
- 2 tbsp vegan butter
- 1 tsp salt

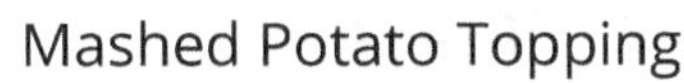

Is the recipe easy to follow?

86. Mushroom and Lentil Shepherd's Pie

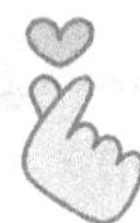

What is the total cooking time, including prep time?

Prep Time : _______________

Cook Time : _______________

Servings : _______________

Ingredients:

- 8 oz rice noodles
- 1 block extra-firm tofu, pressed and cubed
- 2 tbsp coconut oil
- 2 cloves garlic, minced
- 1 cup shredded carrots
- 1 cup bean sprouts
- 1/2 cup chopped green onions
- 1/4 cup chopped cilantro
- 2 tbsp chopped roasted peanuts (optional)

Sauce:
- 3 tbsp tamarind paste
- 2 tbsp coconut aminos or low-sodium soy sauce
- 1 tbsp maple syrup
- 1 tbsp rice vinegar
- 1 tsp ground turmeric
- 1 tsp ground ginger
- 1/4 tsp cayenne pepper
- Salt and pepper to taste

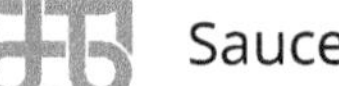

87. Vegan Pad Thai with Tofu

1. Soak the rice noodles in hot water for 15-20 minutes until softened. Drain and set aside.

2. In a small bowl, whisk together all the sauce ingredients. Set aside.

3. In a large skillet or wok, heat the coconut oil over medium-high heat. Add the cubed tofu and cook for 3-4 minutes per side until lightly browned. Remove tofu from the pan and set aside.

4. Add the garlic to the pan and cook for 1 minute until fragrant.

5. Add the softened rice noodles, carrots, bean sprouts, green onions, and the sauce mixture. Toss everything together and cook for 2-3 minutes until the noodles are heated through and the sauce has thickened slightly.

6. Stir the cooked tofu back into the noodle mixture.

7. Remove from heat and stir in the chopped cilantro. Serve the vegan pad thai immediately, garnished with chopped peanuts if desired.

The key anti-inflammatory ingredients in this recipe include:
- Tofu - a good source of plant-based protein and anti-inflammatory isoflavones
- Coconut oil - rich in anti-inflammatory medium-chain triglycerides
- Turmeric - contains the powerful anti-inflammatory compound curcumin
- Ginger - has strong anti-inflammatory properties
- Cayenne pepper - contains capsaicin, which has potent anti-inflammatory effects

What is the total cooking time, including prep time?

Prep Time : ________________

Cook Time : ________________

Servings   : ________________

Ingredients:

- 1 red bell pepper, cut into 1-inch pieces
- 1 yellow bell pepper, cut into 1-inch pieces
- 1 zucchini, cut into 1-inch rounds
- 1 yellow squash, cut into 1-inch rounds
- 1 red onion, cut into 1-inch pieces
- 8 oz cremini mushrooms, halved
- 2 tbsp olive oil
- 2 tsp balsamic vinegar
- 1 tsp dried oregano
- 1 tsp dried basil
- Salt and pepper to taste

Is the recipe easy to follow?

☺   ☹

88. Grilled Vegetable Skewers

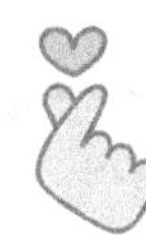

Procedure:

1. Preheat grill to medium-high heat.

2. In a large bowl, combine the chopped bell peppers, zucchini, yellow squash, red onion, and mushrooms.

3. Drizzle the vegetables with the olive oil and balsamic vinegar. Sprinkle with the dried oregano, basil, salt, and pepper. Toss to coat everything evenly.

4. Thread the marinated vegetables onto metal or wooden skewers, leaving a little space between each piece.

5. Grill the vegetable skewers for 12-15 minutes, turning occasionally, until the vegetables are tender and lightly charred.

6. Serve the grilled vegetable skewers immediately, garnished with additional fresh herbs if desired.

Tips:
- Soak wooden skewers in water for 30 minutes before using to prevent them from burning.
- Cut the vegetables into similar-sized pieces so they cook evenly.
- Feel free to use your favorite seasonal vegetables like eggplant, cherry tomatoes, or asparagus.
- Brush the skewers with a bit of olive oil or balsamic glaze during the last few minutes of grilling for extra flavor.
- Serve the grilled vegetable skewers as a main dish, side, or appetizer.

This simple grilled vegetable skewer recipe is a great way to enjoy the fresh flavors of summer produce. The combination of colorful veggies and aromatic herbs makes for a delicious and healthy meal.

What is the total cooking time,
including prep time?

Prep Time : _________________

Cook Time : _________________

Servings   : _________________

Ingredients:

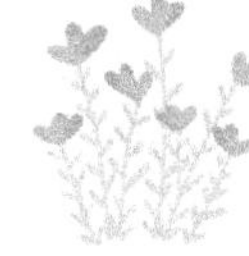

Enchilada Filling:
- 1 tbsp olive oil
- 1 onion, diced
- 3 cloves garlic, minced
- 1 (15 oz) can black beans, drained and rinsed
- 1 cup cooked brown rice
- 1 tsp ground cumin
- 1 tsp chili powder
- 1/2 tsp smoked paprika
- Salt and pepper to taste

Enchilada Sauce:
- 1 (28 oz) can crushed tomatoes
- 2 tbsp tomato paste
- 1 tsp ground cumin
- 1 tsp chili powder
- 1/2 tsp garlic powder
- 1/4 tsp cayenne pepper (optional)
- Salt and pepper to taste

Assembly:
- 8-10 corn tortillas
- 1 cup shredded vegan cheddar cheese (optional)
- Chopped cilantro for garnish

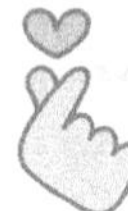

Procedure:

1. Preheat oven to 375°F. Grease a 9x13 inch baking dish.

For the Enchilada Filling:
1. In a large skillet, heat the olive oil over medium heat. Add the onion and sauté for 5 minutes until translucent.
2. Add the garlic and cook for 1 minute until fragrant.
3. Stir in the black beans, cooked rice, cumin, chili powder, and smoked paprika. Season with salt and pepper.
4. Cook for 2-3 minutes, mashing some of the beans slightly, until heated through.

For the Enchilada Sauce:
1. In a medium saucepan, combine the crushed tomatoes, tomato paste, cumin, chili powder, garlic powder, and cayenne (if using).
2. Bring the sauce to a simmer and cook for 5-7 minutes, stirring occasionally, until thickened. Season with salt and pepper.

Assemble the Enchiladas:
1. Spread 1/2 cup of the enchilada sauce in the bottom of the prepared baking dish.
2. Warm the corn tortillas according to package instructions.
3. Spoon about 2-3 tbsp of the black bean filling onto each tortilla. Roll up tightly and place seam-side down in the baking dish.
4. Pour the remaining enchilada sauce over the rolled enchiladas.
5. If using, sprinkle the shredded vegan cheese over the top.
6. Bake for 20-25 minutes until heated through and the cheese is melted.
7. Garnish with chopped cilantro before serving.

Enjoy these delicious and satisfying vegan enchiladas!

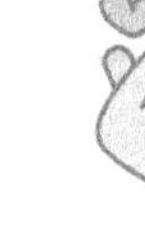

Procedure:

What is the total cooking time,
including prep time?

Prep Time : _______________

Cook Time : _______________

Servings   : _______________

Ingredients:

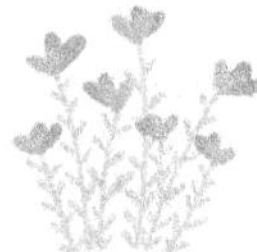

- 4 large portobello mushroom caps, stems removed and chopped
- 2 tbsp olive oil
- 1 onion, diced
- 3 cloves garlic, minced
- 2 cups baby spinach, chopped
- 1 cup cooked quinoa
- 1/4 cup toasted walnuts, chopped
- 2 tbsp nutritional yeast
- 1 tsp dried thyme
- 1/2 tsp ground turmeric
- Salt and pepper to taste

Is the recipe easy to follow?

90. *Stuffed Portobello Mushrooms with Spinach and Quinoa*

1. Preheat oven to 400°F. Lightly grease a baking sheet.

2. Place the portobello mushroom caps gill-side up on the prepared baking sheet. Bake for 10-12 minutes until softened.

3. In a large skillet, heat the olive oil over medium heat. Add the chopped mushroom stems, onion, and garlic. Sauté for 5-7 minutes until onions are translucent.

4. Stir in the spinach and cook for 2-3 minutes until wilted.

5. Remove from heat and stir in the cooked quinoa, walnuts, nutritional yeast, thyme, turmeric, salt, and pepper.

6. Spoon the quinoa-spinach mixture evenly into the baked portobello caps.

7. Return the stuffed mushrooms to the oven and bake for an additional 12-15 minutes until the filling is hot and the mushrooms are tender.

8. Serve the stuffed portobello mushrooms warm.

The key anti-inflammatory ingredients in this recipe include:

- Portobello mushrooms - contain antioxidants and anti-inflammatory compounds
- Spinach - rich in anti-inflammatory vitamins and minerals
- Walnuts - high in anti-inflammatory omega-3 fatty acids
- Turmeric - contains the powerful anti-inflammatory compound curcumin

What is the total cooking time, including prep time?

Prep Time : ________________

Cook Time : ________________

Servings   : ________________

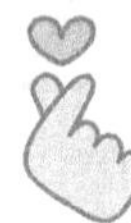

Ingredients:

- 1 lb carrots, peeled and cut into 1-inch pieces
- 1 lb parsnips, peeled and cut into 1-inch pieces
- 1 lb potatoes, peeled and cut into 1-inch pieces
- 1 lb beets, peeled and cut into 1-inch pieces
- 1 red onion, cut into wedges
- 3 tbsp olive oil
- 2 tbsp fresh rosemary, chopped
- 1 tsp salt
- 1/2 tsp black pepper

Is the recipe easy to follow?

☺   ☹

91. Roasted Root Vegetables with Rosemary

Procedure:

1. Preheat the oven to 400°F. Line a large baking sheet with parchment paper.

2. In a large bowl, combine the prepared carrots, parsnips, potatoes, beets, and red onion.

3. Drizzle the vegetables with the olive oil and sprinkle with the chopped rosemary, salt, and pepper. Toss to coat everything evenly.

4. Spread the seasoned vegetables in a single layer on the prepared baking sheet.

5. Roast for 35-45 minutes, stirring halfway, until the vegetables are tender and lightly browned.

6. Serve the roasted root vegetables warm, garnished with additional fresh rosemary if desired.

Tips:
- For even cooking, try to cut the vegetables into similar sized pieces.
- Feel free to use a mix of your favorite root vegetables like sweet potatoes, turnips, or rutabaga.
- Adjust the roasting time as needed depending on the size of your vegetable pieces.
- Toss the roasted veggies with a splash of balsamic vinegar or lemon juice before serving for extra flavor.

This simple roasted root vegetable dish is a great way to enjoy the natural sweetness and earthy flavors of seasonal produce. The rosemary adds a lovely aromatic touch. Serve it as a side dish or as part of a larger plant-based meal.

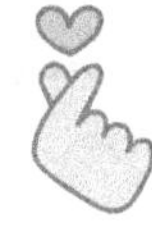

Procedure:

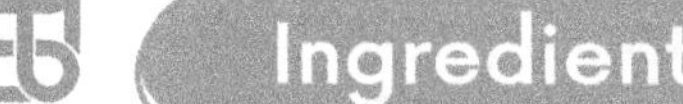 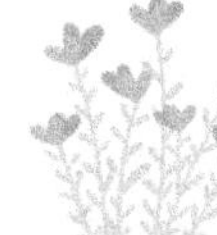

What is the total cooking time, including prep time?

Prep Time : ________________

Cook Time : ________________

Servings : ________________

Ingredients:

- 1 lb Swiss chard, stems removed and leaves chopped
- 2 tbsp olive oil
- 4 cloves garlic, minced
- 1/4 cup low-sodium vegetable broth
- 1 tsp lemon juice
- 1/4 tsp red pepper flakes (optional)
- Salt and pepper to taste

Is the recipe easy to follow?

92. Sautéed Swiss Chard with Garlic

1. In a large skillet or wok, heat the olive oil over medium heat.

2. Add the minced garlic and sauté for 1-2 minutes until fragrant, being careful not to burn.

3. Add the chopped Swiss chard leaves to the pan and toss to coat with the garlic oil.

4. Pour in the vegetable broth and cover the pan. Cook for 3-5 minutes, stirring occasionally, until the chard is wilted and tender.

5. Remove the lid and continue cooking for 1-2 minutes to allow any excess liquid to evaporate.

6. Stir in the lemon juice and red pepper flakes (if using). Season with salt and pepper to taste.

7. Serve the sautéed Swiss chard warm.

The key anti-inflammatory ingredients in this recipe include:

- Swiss chard - packed with antioxidants, vitamins, and minerals that have anti-inflammatory properties
- Olive oil - rich in anti-inflammatory monounsaturated fats
- Garlic - contains sulfur compounds with potent anti-inflammatory effects
- Lemon juice - provides vitamin C and other antioxidants

This makes it a great option for seniors looking to incorporate more anti-inflammatory foods into their diet. The simple preparation allows the natural flavors of the chard and garlic to shine, creating a delicious and nutritious side dish.

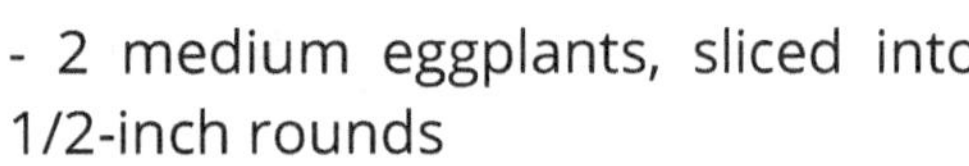

What is the total cooking time,
including prep time?

Prep Time : _______________

Cook Time : _______________

Servings : _______________

Ingredients:

- 2 medium eggplants, sliced into 1/2-inch rounds
- 2 tbsp olive oil, plus more for brushing
- 1 onion, diced
- 3 cloves garlic, minced
- 1 (28 oz) can diced tomatoes
- 2 tbsp tomato paste
- 1 tsp dried oregano
- 1 tsp dried basil
- 1/4 tsp red pepper flakes (optional)
- Salt and pepper to taste
- 1/4 cup grated vegan parmesan cheese (optional)
- Fresh basil leaves for garnish

Is the recipe easy to follow?

93. Baked Eggplant with Tomato Sauce

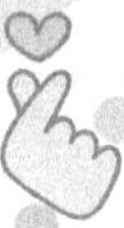

Procedure:

1. Preheat oven to 400°F. Line a baking sheet with parchment paper.

2. Arrange the eggplant slices in a single layer on the prepared baking sheet. Brush both sides lightly with olive oil and season with salt and pepper.

3. Bake for 20-25 minutes, flipping halfway, until the eggplant is tender and lightly browned.

4. In a large skillet, heat 2 tbsp of olive oil over medium heat. Add the onion and sauté for 5-7 minutes until translucent.

5. Add the garlic and cook for 1 minute until fragrant.

6. Stir in the diced tomatoes, tomato paste, oregano, basil, and red pepper flakes (if using). Season with salt and pepper.

7. Simmer the tomato sauce for 10-15 minutes, stirring occasionally, until thickened.

8. Arrange the baked eggplant slices in a baking dish. Pour the tomato sauce over the top and sprinkle with the vegan parmesan cheese, if using.

9. Bake for an additional 15-20 minutes until the cheese is melted and the sauce is bubbly.

10. Garnish with fresh basil leaves before serving.

This makes it a great option for seniors looking to incorporate more anti-inflammatory foods into their diet. The combination of roasted eggplant and flavorful tomato sauce creates a delicious and nourishing meal.

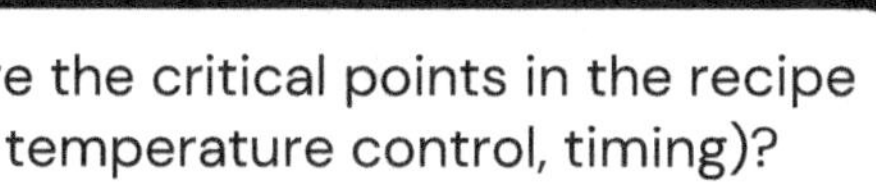

What are the critical points in the recipe (e.g., temperature control, timing)?

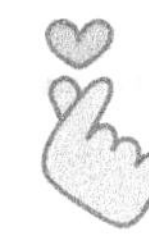

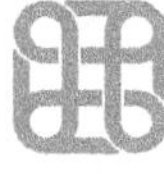

What is the total cooking time, including prep time?

Prep Time : _________________

Cook Time : _________________

Servings : _________________

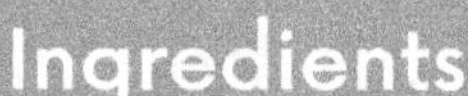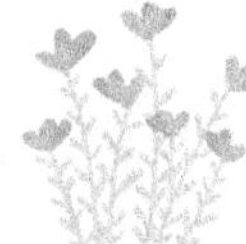

Ingredients:

- 4 ears of corn, husks and silk removed
- 2 tbsp olive oil
- 1 lime, cut into wedges
- 1/4 cup chopped fresh cilantro (optional)
- Salt and pepper to taste

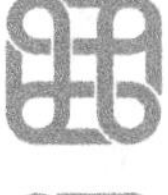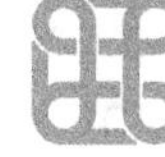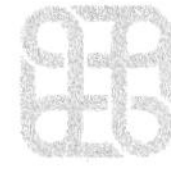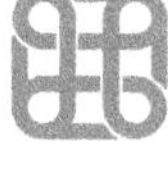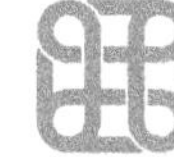

Is the recipe easy to follow?

94. *Grilled Corn on the Cob with Lime*

1. Preheat your grill to medium-high heat.

2. Brush the corn cobs all over with the olive oil, making sure to coat them evenly.

3. Place the oiled corn cobs directly on the grill grates. Grill for 12-15 minutes, rotating the cobs occasionally, until the kernels are tender and lightly charred.

4. Remove the grilled corn from the grill and transfer to a serving platter.

5. Squeeze the lime wedges over the hot corn, allowing the juice to drizzle over the kernels.

6. If using, sprinkle the chopped cilantro over the top of the grilled corn.

7. Season with salt and pepper to taste. Serve the grilled corn on the cob immediately, with extra lime wedges on the side.

- Soak the corn cobs in water for 30 minutes before grilling to help prevent the husks from burning.
- For extra flavor, rub the corn with a mixture of olive oil, chili powder, garlic powder, and lime zest before grilling.
- Try different herb combinations, such as basil, oregano, or parsley, instead of or in addition to the cilantro.
- Serve the grilled corn as a side dish or as part of a larger grilled meal.

The smoky, charred flavor of the grilled corn paired with the bright, tangy lime juice makes for a delicious and simple summer side dish. The optional cilantro adds a fresh, herbal note. Enjoy this grilled corn on the cob as a tasty accompaniment to your favorite plant-based main courses.

What are the critical points in the recipe (e.g., temperature control, timing)?

What is the total cooking time, including prep time?

Prep Time : ___________________

Cook Time : ___________________

Servings   : ___________________

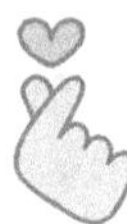

Ingredients:

- 1 head of cauliflower, cut into florets
- 2 tbsp olive oil
- 1 tsp ground turmeric
- 1 tsp ground cumin
- 1/2 tsp garlic powder
- 1/4 tsp cayenne pepper (optional)
- 1/2 tsp salt
- 1/4 tsp black pepper
- 2 tbsp chopped fresh parsley (for garnish)

Is the recipe easy to follow?

🙂   🙁

95. Roasted Cauliflower with Turmeric

Procedure:

1. Preheat the oven to 400°F. Line a large baking sheet with parchment paper.

2. In a large bowl, toss the cauliflower florets with the olive oil, turmeric, cumin, garlic powder, cayenne (if using), salt, and black pepper until the cauliflower is evenly coated.

3. Spread the seasoned cauliflower in a single layer on the prepared baking sheet.

4. Roast for 20-25 minutes, flipping the cauliflower halfway, until the florets are tender and lightly browned.

5. Remove the roasted cauliflower from the oven and transfer to a serving dish.

6. Sprinkle the chopped fresh parsley over the top.

7. Serve the roasted cauliflower warm.

Tips:
- Cut the cauliflower florets into similar-sized pieces so they cook evenly.
- Adjust the roasting time based on the size of your cauliflower pieces.
- For extra crispiness, broil the cauliflower for the last 2-3 minutes of cooking.
- Toss the roasted cauliflower with a squeeze of lemon juice or a drizzle of tahini sauce before serving.
- Sprinkle with toasted nuts or seeds for added crunch.

The turmeric not only gives the cauliflower a beautiful golden color, but also provides anti-inflammatory benefits. Paired with the warmth of cumin and the kick of cayenne, this roasted cauliflower dish is full of flavor. Enjoy it as a side or as part of a larger plant-based meal.

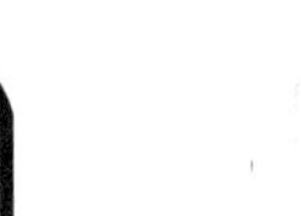

Procedure:

What is the total cooking time, including prep time?

Prep Time : _______________

Cook Time : _______________

Servings : _______________

Ingredients:

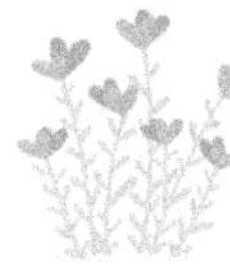

- 1 lb green beans, trimmed
- 2 tbsp olive oil
- 1/4 cup sliced almonds
- 2 cloves garlic, minced
- 1 tbsp lemon juice
- 1 tsp Dijon mustard
- 1/4 tsp salt
- 1/4 tsp black pepper

Is the recipe easy to follow?

96. Steamed Green Beans with Almonds

1. Fill a large pot with 1-2 inches of water and bring to a boil. Place a steamer basket in the pot.

2. Add the trimmed green beans to the steamer basket. Cover and steam for 5-7 minutes, until the beans are tender-crisp.

3. Meanwhile, in a small skillet, toast the sliced almonds over medium heat for 2-3 minutes, stirring frequently, until lightly golden brown. Transfer the toasted almonds to a plate and set aside.

4. In a small bowl, whisk together the olive oil, lemon juice, Dijon mustard, salt, and pepper.

5. Once the green beans are steamed, transfer them to a serving bowl. Drizzle the lemon-mustard dressing over the beans and toss to coat.

6. Sprinkle the toasted almond slices over the dressed green beans.

7. Serve the steamed green beans with almonds warm or at room temperature.

Tips:
- For extra flavor, add a pinch of red pepper flakes or some chopped fresh herbs to the dressing.
- Substitute slivered almonds or chopped walnuts if preferred.
- Blanch the green beans in boiling water for 2-3 minutes instead of steaming, if desired.
- Toss the beans with the dressing while they are still warm so the flavors meld together.

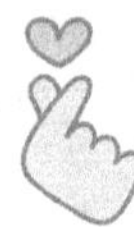

What are the critical points in the recipe (e.g., temperature control, timing)?

What is the total cooking time, including prep time?

Prep Time : _______________

Cook Time : _______________

Servings : _______________

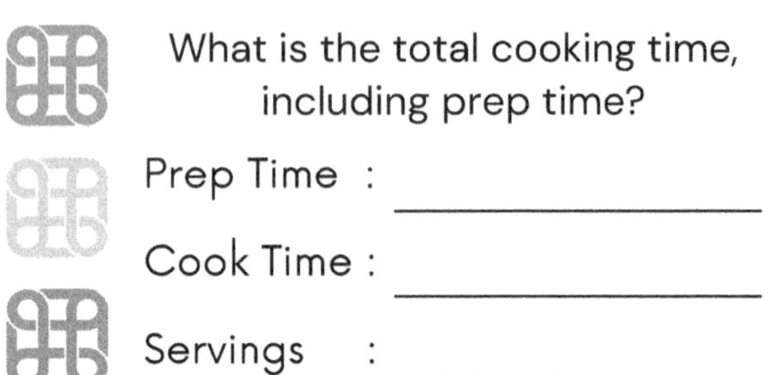

Ingredients:

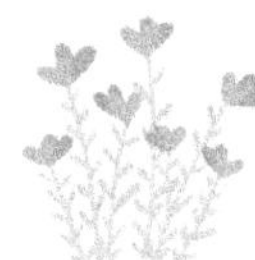

- 1 lb baby bok choy, washed and cut into 1-inch pieces
- 2 tbsp sesame oil
- 2 tbsp low-sodium soy sauce or tamari
- 1 tbsp rice vinegar
- 1 tbsp maple syrup
- 2 tsp grated fresh ginger
- 2 cloves garlic, minced
- 1/4 tsp red pepper flakes (optional)
- Salt and pepper to taste
- Toasted sesame seeds for garnish (optional)

Is the recipe easy to follow?

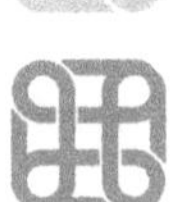
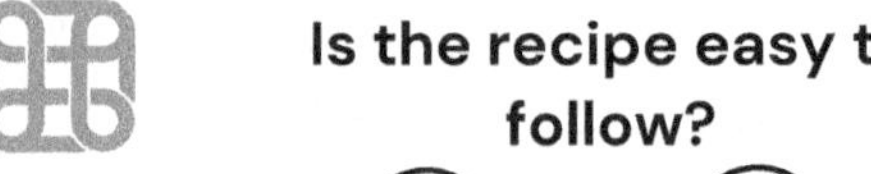

97. Sautéed Bok Choy with Ginger

1. In a large skillet or wok, heat the sesame oil over medium-high heat.

2. Add the chopped bok choy and sauté for 2-3 minutes, stirring frequently, until the leaves start to wilt.

3. In a small bowl, whisk together the soy sauce, rice vinegar, maple syrup, grated ginger, and garlic.

4. Pour the sauce mixture into the skillet with the bok choy. Toss everything together and continue cooking for 2-3 minutes, until the bok choy is tender-crisp.

5. If using, sprinkle in the red pepper flakes and season with salt and pepper to taste.

6. Remove from heat and transfer the sautéed bok choy to a serving dish. Garnish with toasted sesame seeds, if desired.

Serve the bok choy warm as a side dish or over steamed rice for a complete meal.

Tips:
- Look for baby bok choy, which has a more tender texture than full-sized bok choy.
- Adjust the cooking time based on the size and maturity of your bok choy.
- For extra crunch, add some toasted nuts or seeds to the dish.
- Substitute the maple syrup with honey or agave nectar if preferred.

This simple sautéed bok choy with ginger is a quick and flavorful way to enjoy this nutritious Chinese green. The ginger and garlic provide a nice aromatic base, while the soy sauce and rice vinegar add a savory-tangy balance.

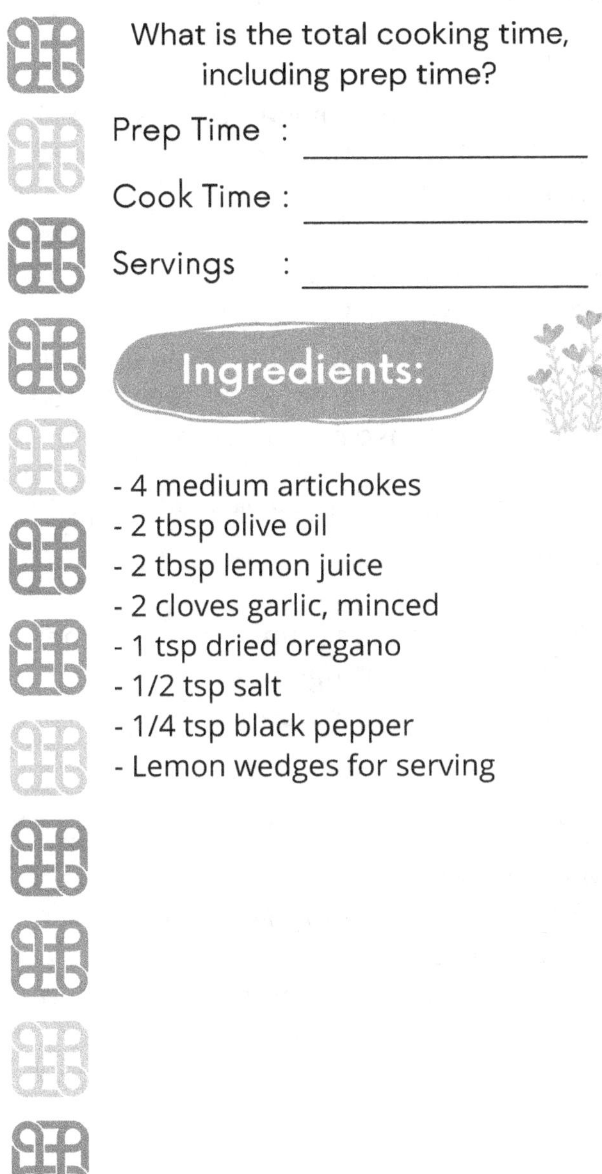

What is the total cooking time, including prep time?

Prep Time : _______________

Cook Time : _______________

Servings   : _______________

Ingredients:

- 4 medium artichokes
- 2 tbsp olive oil
- 2 tbsp lemon juice
- 2 cloves garlic, minced
- 1 tsp dried oregano
- 1/2 tsp salt
- 1/4 tsp black pepper
- Lemon wedges for serving

Is the recipe easy to follow?

98. Roasted Artichokes with Lemon

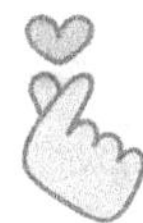

Procedure:

1. Preheat the oven to 400°F. Line a baking sheet with parchment paper.

2. Prepare the artichokes:
- Trim the stems of the artichokes, leaving about 1 inch.
- Use kitchen shears to snip off the thorny tips of the outer leaves.
- Cut the artichokes in half lengthwise.
- Use a spoon to scoop out the fuzzy choke and any purple leaves in the center.

3. In a small bowl, whisk together the olive oil, lemon juice, garlic, oregano, salt, and pepper.

4. Place the artichoke halves cut-side up on the prepared baking sheet. Brush the artichokes generously with the lemon-garlic mixture, making sure to get it in between the leaves.

5. Roast the artichokes for 30-40 minutes, basting with the pan juices halfway, until the leaves are tender and the bottoms are browned.

6. Serve the roasted artichokes warm, with lemon wedges on the side for squeezing over the top.

Tips:
- Look for artichokes that are heavy for their size with tightly packed leaves.
- Rub the cut surfaces with lemon juice to prevent browning.
- Adjust the roasting time based on the size of your artichokes.
- Dip the leaves in a flavorful dipping sauce like aioli, pesto, or balsamic reduction.

Roasting brings out the natural sweetness of artichokes and the lemon-garlic seasoning adds a bright, savory flavor. This simple preparation makes for a delicious and elegant side dish or appetizer.

What are the critical points in the recipe (e.g., temperature control, timing)?

Procedure:

1. Preheat the oven to 375°F. Line a baking sheet with parchment paper.

2. Slice the tops off the tomatoes and scoop out the seeds and pulp, leaving a hollow shell. Finely chop the scooped out tomato flesh.

3. In a medium bowl, combine the chopped tomato flesh, cooked quinoa, parsley, basil, chives, garlic, olive oil, balsamic vinegar, salt, and pepper. Mix well.

4. Stuff the quinoa mixture evenly into the hollowed-out tomato shells.

5. If using, sprinkle the tops of the stuffed tomatoes with the panko breadcrumbs.

6. Place the stuffed tomatoes on the prepared baking sheet.

7. Bake for 20-25 minutes, until the tomatoes are softened and the filling is heated through. Serve the stuffed tomatoes warm.

Tips:
- Choose firm, ripe tomatoes that can hold their shape when stuffed.
- For extra flavor, try adding grated Parmesan cheese or crumbled feta to the quinoa filling.
- Swap in different fresh herbs like oregano, thyme, or cilantro based on your preferences.
- Stuff the tomatoes ahead of time and refrigerate until ready to bake.
- Serve the stuffed tomatoes as a main dish, side, or appetizer.

These colorful and flavorful stuffed tomatoes make a delightful plant-based meal or side. The combination of juicy tomatoes, nutty quinoa, and fresh herbs creates a delicious and satisfying dish.

What is the total cooking time, including prep time?

Prep Time : _______________

Cook Time : _______________

Servings   : _______________

Ingredients:

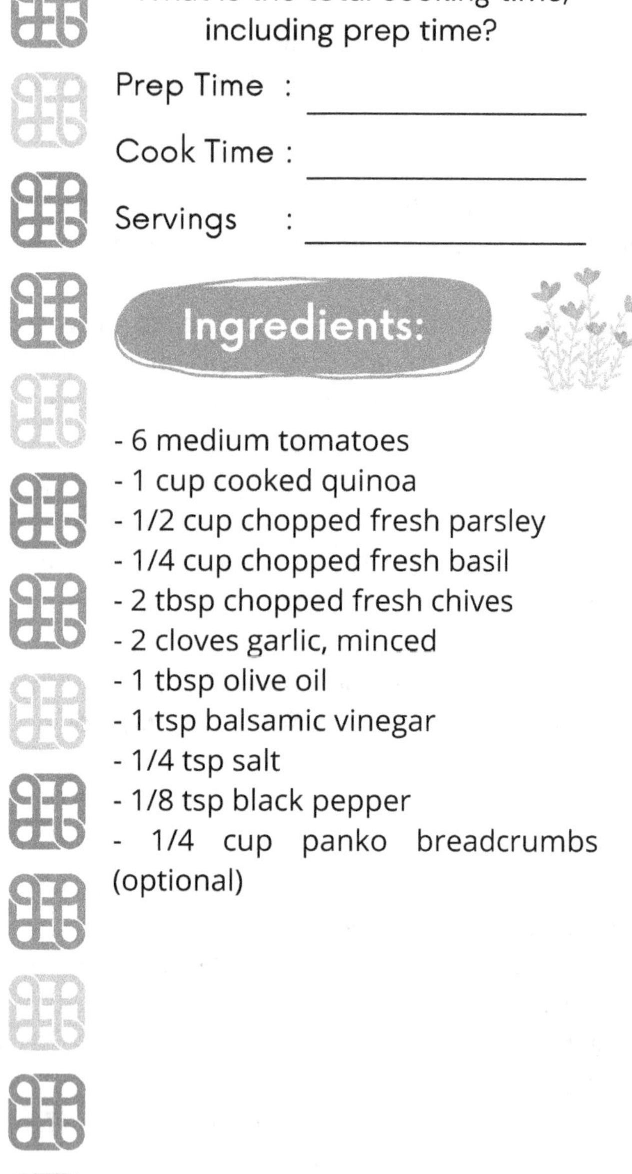

- 6 medium tomatoes
- 1 cup cooked quinoa
- 1/2 cup chopped fresh parsley
- 1/4 cup chopped fresh basil
- 2 tbsp chopped fresh chives
- 2 cloves garlic, minced
- 1 tbsp olive oil
- 1 tsp balsamic vinegar
- 1/4 tsp salt
- 1/8 tsp black pepper
- 1/4 cup panko breadcrumbs (optional)

Is the recipe easy to follow?

99. Stuffed Tomatoes with Quinoa and Herbs

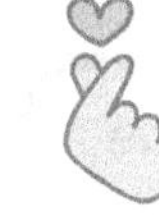

What is the total cooking time,
including prep time?

Prep Time : ___________________

Cook Time : ___________________

Servings   : ___________________

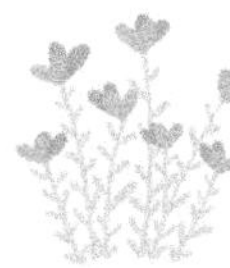

Ingredients:

- 1 lb Brussels sprouts, trimmed and halved
- 2 tbsp olive oil
- 2 tbsp maple syrup
- 1 tsp Dijon mustard
- 1/2 tsp salt
- 1/4 tsp black pepper
- 1/2 cup pecan halves

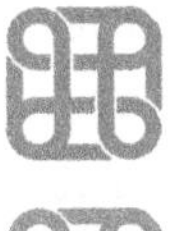
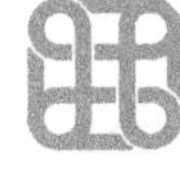
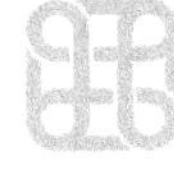
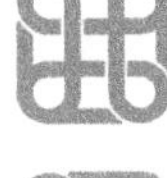
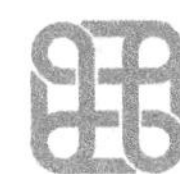

**Is the recipe easy to
follow?**

*100. Caramelized Brussels Sprouts
with Pecans*

1. Preheat the oven to 400°F. Line a large baking sheet with parchment paper.

2. In a large bowl, toss the Brussels sprout halves with the olive oil, maple syrup, Dijon mustard, salt, and pepper until evenly coated.

3. Spread the seasoned Brussels sprouts in a single layer on the prepared baking sheet.

4. Roast for 20-25 minutes, stirring halfway, until the Brussels sprouts are tender and caramelized.

5. During the last 5 minutes of roasting, add the pecan halves to the baking sheet and continue cooking until the pecans are lightly toasted.

6. Remove the pan from the oven and transfer the caramelized Brussels sprouts and pecans to a serving dish.

7. Serve the Brussels sprouts warm, garnished with any remaining toasted pecans.

Tips:
- For even cooking, make sure the Brussels sprouts are cut in half and spread in a single layer on the baking sheet.
- Adjust the roasting time based on the size of your Brussels sprouts. Smaller sprouts may cook faster.
- Try adding a sprinkle of red pepper flakes or a squeeze of lemon juice for extra flavor.
- Substitute walnuts or almonds for the pecans if desired.
- Serve the caramelized Brussels sprouts as a side dish or toss them with cooked pasta or grains for a main meal.

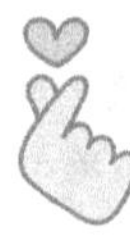

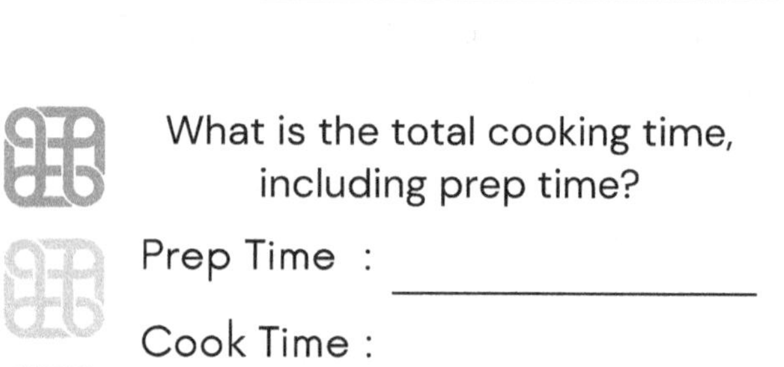

What is the total cooking time, including prep time?

Prep Time : _______________

Cook Time : _______________

Servings   : _______________

Ingredients:

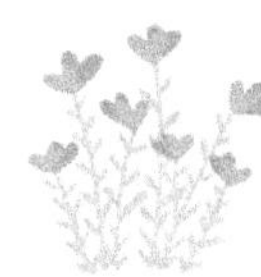

- 1 cup uncooked farro, rinsed
- 2 cups low-sodium vegetable broth
- 1 pint cherry tomatoes, halved
- 1 cup fresh basil leaves, chopped
- 1/2 cup diced cucumber
- 1/4 cup diced red onion
- 2 tbsp olive oil
- 2 tbsp balsamic vinegar
- 1 tsp Dijon mustard
- 1 tsp honey
- 1/4 tsp ground turmeric
- Salt and pepper to taste

Is the recipe easy to follow?

101. Farro Salad with Cherry Tomatoes and Basil

1. In a medium saucepan, combine the farro and vegetable broth. Bring to a boil, then reduce heat and simmer for 20-25 minutes, until the farro is tender. Drain any excess liquid and let cool.

2. In a large bowl, combine the cooked farro, cherry tomatoes, basil, cucumber, and red onion.

3. In a small bowl, whisk together the olive oil, balsamic vinegar, Dijon mustard, honey, and turmeric. Season with salt and pepper.

4. Pour the dressing over the farro salad and toss gently to coat.

5. Cover and refrigerate the salad for at least 30 minutes to allow the flavors to meld.

6. Serve the farro salad chilled or at room temperature.

The key anti-inflammatory ingredients in this recipe include:

- Farro - a whole grain that is high in fiber and antioxidants
- Cherry tomatoes - rich in the antioxidant lycopene
- Basil - contains anti-inflammatory compounds
- Olive oil - a source of anti-inflammatory monounsaturated fats
- Turmeric - contains the powerful anti-inflammatory compound curcumin

This makes it a great option for seniors looking to incorporate more anti-inflammatory foods into their diet. The combination of whole grains, fresh produce, and healthy fats provides a nourishing and flavorful salad that can be enjoyed as a main dish or side.

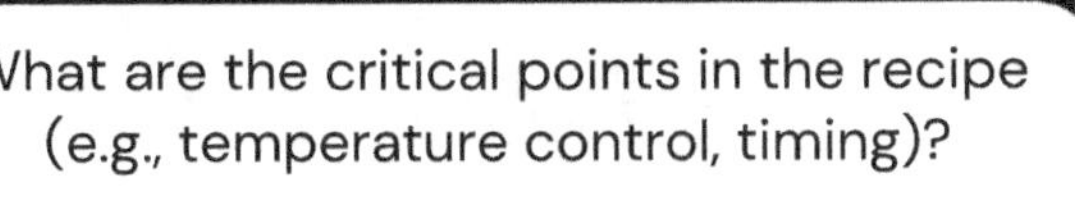 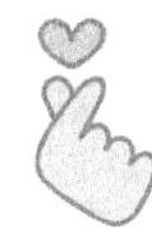

Procedure:

1. In a large bowl, combine the drained and rinsed black beans, drained corn, diced bell pepper, halved cherry tomatoes, and diced red onion.

2. Add the chopped cilantro to the vegetable mixture.

3. In a small bowl, whisk together the olive oil, lime juice, cumin, chili powder, salt, and black pepper.

4. Pour the dressing over the black bean and corn salad and toss gently to coat.

5. Cover and refrigerate the salad for at least 30 minutes to allow the flavors to meld.

6. Serve chilled or at room temperature.

Tips:
- Use fresh or frozen corn kernels instead of canned, if preferred.
- Add diced avocado or crumbled feta cheese for extra flavor and creaminess.
- For a spicier salad, add a finely diced jalapeño or a pinch of cayenne pepper.
- Swap the cilantro for parsley or green onions if desired.
- Serve the black bean and corn salad as a side dish, or enjoy it as a main course over a bed of greens.

This vibrant and refreshing black bean and corn salad is packed with flavor and nutrition. The combination of protein-rich black beans, sweet corn, crunchy vegetables, and a zesty lime-cumin dressing makes it a delicious and versatile dish.

What is the total cooking time, including prep time?

Prep Time : ___________________

Cook Time : ___________________

Servings   : ___________________

Ingredients:

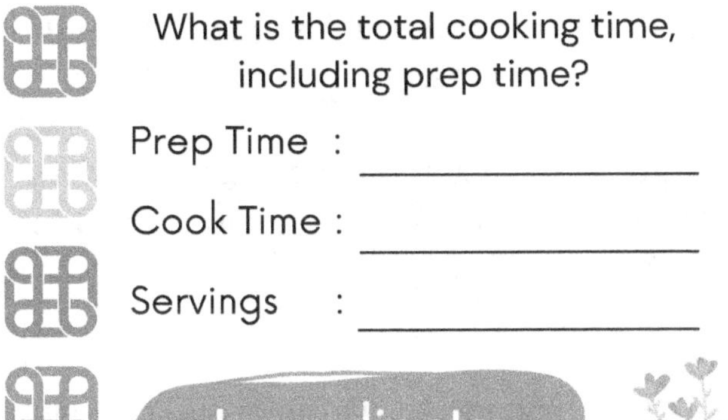 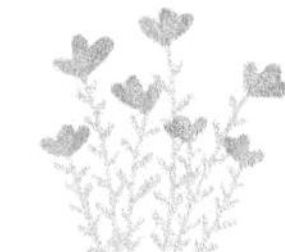

- 1 (15 oz) can black beans, drained and rinsed
- 1 (15 oz) can corn, drained
- 1 red bell pepper, diced
- 1 cup cherry tomatoes, halved
- 1/2 red onion, diced
- 1/4 cup chopped fresh cilantro
- 2 tbsp olive oil
- 2 tbsp lime juice
- 1 tsp ground cumin
- 1/2 tsp chili powder
- 1/4 tsp salt
- 1/4 tsp black pepper

Is the recipe easy to follow?

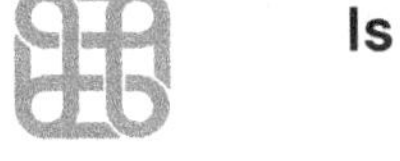  

102. Black Bean and Corn Salad

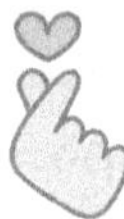

What is the total cooking time, including prep time?

Prep Time : _______________

Cook Time : _______________

Servings : _______________

Ingredients:

- 1 cup uncooked quinoa, rinsed
- 2 cups low-sodium vegetable broth
- 1 lb mixed vegetables (such as sweet potatoes, bell peppers, zucchini, and onions), cut into 1-inch pieces
- 2 tbsp olive oil
- 1 tsp ground turmeric
- 1 tsp ground cumin
- 1/2 tsp garlic powder
- 1/4 tsp cayenne pepper (optional)
- Salt and pepper to taste
- 2 tbsp chopped fresh parsley
- 2 tbsp chopped fresh basil

Is the recipe easy to follow?

103. *Quinoa with Roasted Vegetables*

1. Preheat the oven to 400°F. Line a large baking sheet with parchment paper.

2. In a medium saucepan, combine the quinoa and vegetable broth. Bring to a boil, then reduce heat and simmer for 15-20 minutes, until the quinoa is tender and the liquid is absorbed. Fluff with a fork and set aside.

3. In a large bowl, toss the chopped vegetables with the olive oil, turmeric, cumin, garlic powder, and cayenne (if using). Season with salt and pepper.

4. Spread the seasoned vegetables in a single layer on the prepared baking sheet.

5. Roast the vegetables for 20-25 minutes, stirring halfway, until they are tender and lightly browned.

6. In a large bowl, combine the cooked quinoa and roasted vegetables. Stir in the chopped parsley and basil.

7. Serve the quinoa and roasted vegetable dish warm.

The key anti-inflammatory ingredients in this recipe include:

- Quinoa - a nutrient-dense whole grain
- Sweet potatoes - high in anti-inflammatory beta-carotene
- Olive oil - rich in anti-inflammatory monounsaturated fats
- Turmeric - contains the powerful anti-inflammatory compound curcumin
- Herbs like parsley and basil - provide antioxidants and anti-inflammatory benefits

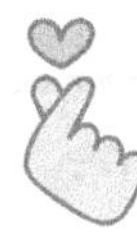

What is the total cooking time, including prep time?

Prep Time : _______________

Cook Time : _______________

Servings : _______________

Ingredients:

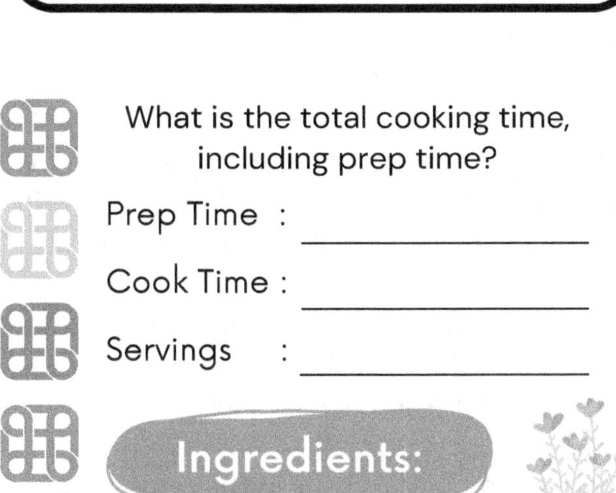

- 1 cup brown or green lentlls, rinsed
- 3 cups low-sodium vegetable broth
- 1 tbsp olive oil
- 1 onion, diced
- 3 cloves garlic, minced
- 1 cup diced carrots
- 1 cup diced celery
- 1 cup diced bell pepper
- 1 tsp ground turmeric
- 1 tsp ground cumin
- 1 tsp dried thyme
- 1/2 tsp ground coriander
- Salt and pepper to taste
- 1/4 cup chopped fresh parsley
- Lemon wedges for serving

Is the recipe easy to follow?

104. Lentil and Vegetable Pilaf

1. In a medium saucepan, combine the lentils and vegetable broth. Bring to a boil, then reduce heat and simmer for 20-25 minutes, until the lentils are tender. Drain any excess liquid and set aside.

2. In a large skillet or wok, heat the olive oil over medium heat. Add the onion and sauté for 5 minutes until translucent.

3. Add the garlic, carrots, celery, and bell pepper. Sauté for 7-10 minutes, stirring occasionally, until the vegetables are tender.

4. Stir in the cooked lentils, turmeric, cumin, thyme, and coriander. Season with salt and pepper to taste.

5. Cook for an additional 5 minutes, allowing the flavors to meld together.

6. Remove from heat and stir in the chopped parsley. Serve the lentil and vegetable pilaf warm, with lemon wedges on the side.

The key anti-inflammatory ingredients in this recipe include:
- Lentils - high in fiber, protein, and anti-inflammatory nutrients
- Turmeric - contains the powerful anti-inflammatory compound curcumin
- Olive oil - rich in anti-inflammatory monounsaturated fats
- Vegetables like carrots, celery, and bell peppers - packed with antioxidants and anti-inflammatory vitamins

This makes it a great option for seniors looking to incorporate more anti-inflammatory foods into their diet. The combination of hearty lentils, aromatic spices, and fresh vegetables creates a nourishing and flavorful one-dish meal.

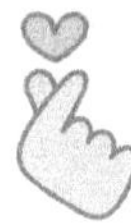

What are the critical points in the recipe (e.g., temperature control, timing)?

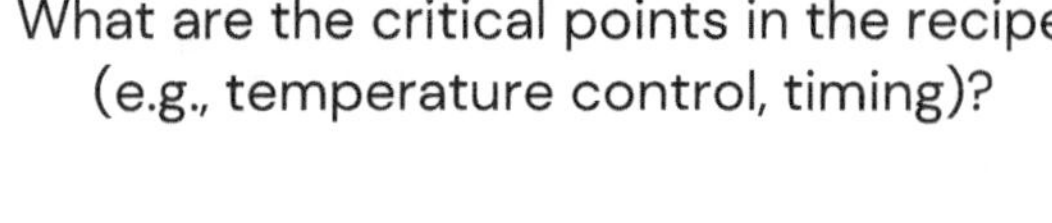

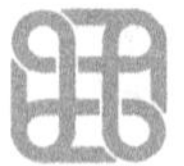 What is the total cooking time, including prep time?

Prep Time : _______________

Cook Time : _______________

Servings : _______________

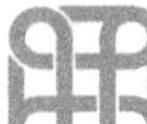

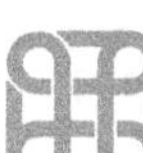

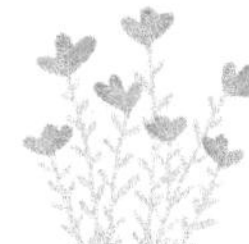

Ingredients:

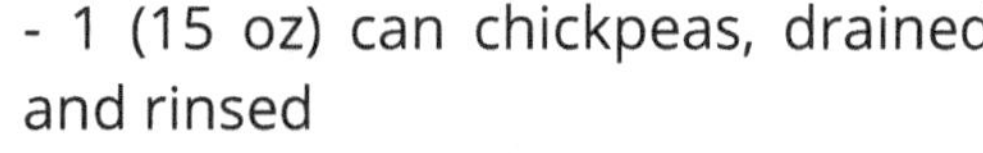

- 2 tbsp olive oil
- 1 onion, diced
- 3 cloves garlic, minced
- 1 (15 oz) can chickpeas, drained and rinsed
- 1 tsp ground cumin
- 1 tsp ground turmeric
- 1/2 tsp smoked paprika
- 1/4 tsp cayenne pepper (optional)
- 5 oz baby spinach
- 1/4 cup low-sodium vegetable broth
- 1 tbsp lemon juice
- Salt and pepper to taste
- Chopped fresh parsley for garnish

Is the recipe easy to follow?

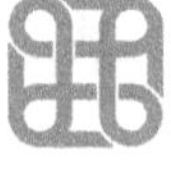

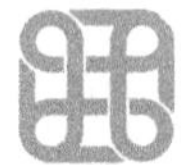

105. Chickpea and Spinach Sauté

1. In a large skillet, heat the olive oil over medium heat. Add the diced onion and sauté for 5 minutes until translucent.

2. Stir in the minced garlic and cook for 1 minute until fragrant.

3. Add the drained and rinsed chickpeas, cumin, turmeric, smoked paprika, and cayenne (if using). Toss to coat the chickpeas in the spices.

4. Add the baby spinach and vegetable broth to the skillet. Cook for 2-3 minutes, stirring frequently, until the spinach is wilted.

5. Remove from heat and stir in the lemon juice. Season with salt and pepper to taste.

6. Serve the chickpea and spinach sauté warm, garnished with chopped fresh parsley.

The key anti-inflammatory ingredients in this recipe include:

- Chickpeas - a good source of plant-based protein and fiber
- Olive oil - rich in anti-inflammatory monounsaturated fats
- Turmeric - contains the powerful anti-inflammatory compound curcumin
- Spinach - packed with antioxidants and anti-inflammatory nutrients
- Lemon juice - provides vitamin C and other anti-inflammatory benefits

This makes it a great option for seniors looking to incorporate more anti-inflammatory foods into their diet. The combination of protein-rich chickpeas, nutrient-dense spinach, and aromatic spices creates a simple yet flavorful plant-based dish.

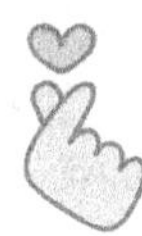

What is the total cooking time,
including prep time?

Prep Time : _________________

Cook Time : _________________

Servings   : _________________

Ingredients:

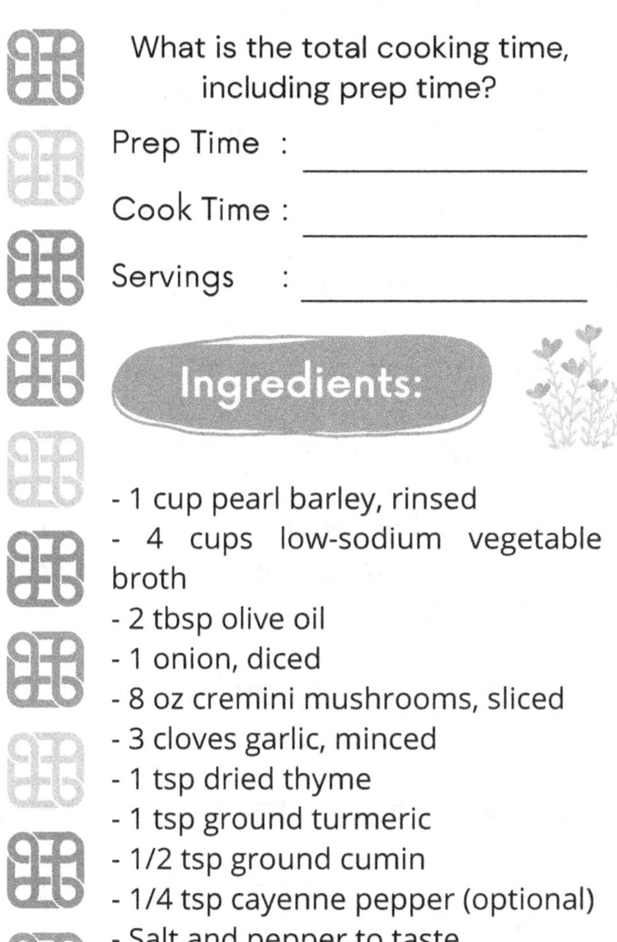

- 1 cup pearl barley, rinsed
- 4 cups low-sodium vegetable broth
- 2 tbsp olive oil
- 1 onion, diced
- 8 oz cremini mushrooms, sliced
- 3 cloves garlic, minced
- 1 tsp dried thyme
- 1 tsp ground turmeric
- 1/2 tsp ground cumin
- 1/4 tsp cayenne pepper (optional)
- Salt and pepper to taste
- 2 tbsp chopped fresh parsley
- 2 tbsp grated Parmesan cheese (optional)

Is the recipe easy to follow?

106. Barley and Mushroom Risotto

1. In a medium saucepan, combine the barley and vegetable broth. Bring to a boil, then reduce heat and simmer for 25-30 minutes, until the barley is tender. Drain any excess liquid and set aside.

2. In a large skillet, heat the olive oil over medium heat. Add the diced onion and sauté for 5 minutes until translucent.

3. Add the sliced mushrooms and continue cooking for 5-7 minutes, until the mushrooms are softened.

4. Stir in the minced garlic, thyme, turmeric, cumin, and cayenne (if using). Season with salt and pepper.

5. Add the cooked barley to the skillet and stir to combine. Cook for an additional 2-3 minutes, allowing the flavors to meld.

6. Remove from heat and stir in the chopped parsley.

7. Serve the barley and mushroom risotto warm, garnished with the optional Parmesan cheese.

The key anti-inflammatory ingredients in this recipe include:

- Barley - a whole grain that is high in fiber and antioxidants
- Mushrooms - contain anti-inflammatory compounds
- Olive oil - rich in anti-inflammatory monounsaturated fats
- Turmeric - contains the powerful anti-inflammatory compound curcumin
- Herbs like thyme and parsley - provide antioxidants and anti-inflammatory benefits

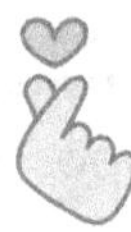

Procedure:

1. Cook the brown rice according to package instructions. Set aside.

2. In a large skillet, heat the olive oil over medium heat. Add the diced onion and sauté for 5 minutes until translucent.

3. Stir in the minced garlic and jalapeño (if using). Cook for 1 minute until fragrant.

4. Add the drained and rinsed black beans, cumin, chili powder, oregano, turmeric, and cayenne (if using). Season with salt and pepper.

5. Reduce heat to low and simmer the black bean mixture for 10-15 minutes, stirring occasionally, until the flavors have melded.

6. Serve the spicy black beans over the cooked brown rice. Garnish with chopped cilantro and serve with lime wedges.

The key anti-inflammatory ingredients in this recipe include:

- Brown rice - a whole grain that is high in fiber and antioxidants
- Black beans - a good source of plant-based protein and fiber
- Olive oil - rich in anti-inflammatory monounsaturated fats
- Turmeric - contains the powerful anti-inflammatory compound curcumin
- Spices like cumin, chili powder, and cayenne - have potent anti-inflammatory properties
- Cilantro - provides antioxidants and anti-inflammatory benefits

---

What is the total cooking time, including prep time?

Prep Time : _________________

Cook Time : _________________

Servings   : _________________

Ingredients:

- 1 cup uncooked brown rice
- 2 (15 oz) cans black beans, drained and rinsed
- 2 tbsp olive oil
- 1 onion, diced
- 3 cloves garlic, minced
- 1 jalapeño, seeded and minced (optional)
- 1 tsp ground cumin
- 1 tsp chili powder
- 1 tsp dried oregano
- 1/2 tsp ground turmeric
- 1/4 tsp cayenne pepper (optional)
- Salt and pepper to taste
- Chopped cilantro for garnish
- Lime wedges for serving

Is the recipe easy to follow?

107. *Spicy Black Beans with Brown Rice*

What are the critical points in the recipe (e.g., temperature control, timing)?

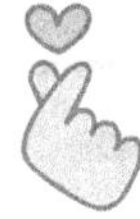

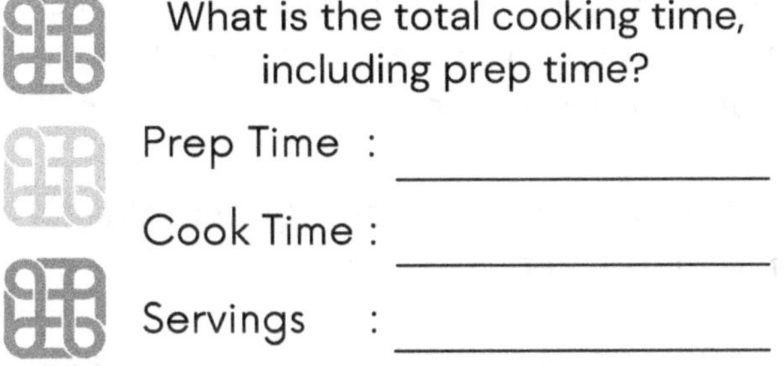

What is the total cooking time, including prep time?

Prep Time : _________________

Cook Time : _________________

Servings   : _________________

Ingredients:

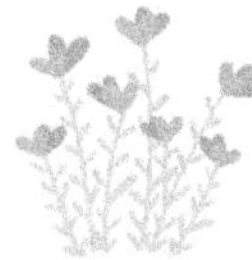

- 1 tablespoon olive oil
- 1 onion, diced
- 3 cloves garlic, minced
- 1 bunch kale, stems removed and leaves chopped
- 1 (15 oz) can white beans, drained and rinsed
- 1/4 cup vegetable broth
- 1 teaspoon lemon juice
- Salt and pepper to taste

Is the recipe easy to follow?

108. White Bean and Kale Sauté

1. In a large skillet, heat the olive oil over medium heat. Add the onion and sauté for 5 minutes until translucent.

2. Add the garlic and sauté for 1 minute until fragrant.

3. Add the chopped kale and sauté for 3-5 minutes, until the kale is wilted and tender.

4. Stir in the white beans and vegetable broth. Simmer for 5 minutes, allowing the flavors to meld.

5. Remove from heat and stir in the lemon juice. Season with salt and pepper to taste.

This dish is packed with anti-inflammatory ingredients like kale, which is high in antioxidants and vitamins A, C, and K. The white beans provide plant-based protein and fiber, which can help support healthy digestion and blood sugar levels. The olive oil and lemon juice also have anti-inflammatory properties.

This sauté makes a great side dish or can be served as a main course over whole grains. It's a simple, nutritious meal that may be beneficial for seniors looking to reduce inflammation.

What are the critical points in the recipe (e.g., temperature control, timing)?

What is the total cooking time, including prep time?

Prep Time : ___________________

Cook Time : ___________________

Servings   : ___________________

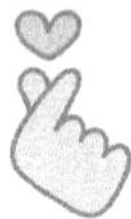

Ingredients:

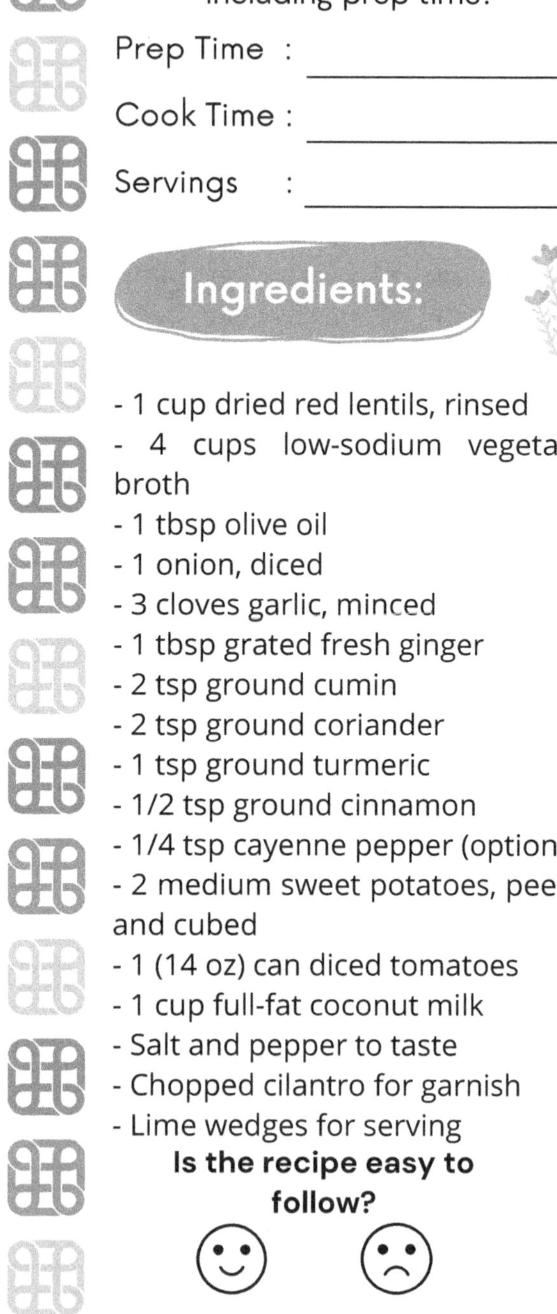

- 1 cup dried red lentils, rinsed
- 4 cups low-sodium vegetable broth
- 1 tbsp olive oil
- 1 onion, diced
- 3 cloves garlic, minced
- 1 tbsp grated fresh ginger
- 2 tsp ground cumin
- 2 tsp ground coriander
- 1 tsp ground turmeric
- 1/2 tsp ground cinnamon
- 1/4 tsp cayenne pepper (optional)
- 2 medium sweet potatoes, peeled and cubed
- 1 (14 oz) can diced tomatoes
- 1 cup full-fat coconut milk
- Salt and pepper to taste
- Chopped cilantro for garnish
- Lime wedges for serving

Is the recipe easy to follow?

:)   :(

109. Lentil and Sweet Potato Curry

Procedure:

1. In a large pot, combine the rinsed lentils and vegetable broth. Bring to a boil, then reduce heat and simmer for 15-20 minutes, until the lentils are tender. Drain any excess liquid and set aside.

2. In the same pot, heat the olive oil over medium heat. Add the diced onion and sauté for 5 minutes until translucent.

3. Stir in the minced garlic and grated ginger. Cook for 1 minute until fragrant.

4. Add the cumin, coriander, turmeric, cinnamon, and cayenne (if using). Stir to coat the onion mixture in the spices.

5. Add the cubed sweet potatoes, diced tomatoes, and coconut milk. Bring to a simmer and cook for 15-20 minutes, until the sweet potatoes are tender.

6. Stir the cooked lentils into the curry. Season with salt and pepper to taste.

7. Serve the lentil and sweet potato curry warm, garnished with chopped cilantro. Provide lime wedges on the side.

The key anti-inflammatory ingredients in this recipe include:

- Lentils - a good source of plant-based protein and fiber
- Sweet potatoes - high in anti-inflammatory beta-carotene
- Olive oil - rich in anti-inflammatory monounsaturated fats
- Turmeric - contains the powerful anti-inflammatory compound curcumin
- Ginger - has strong anti-inflammatory properties

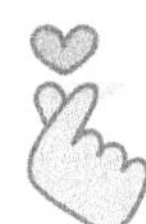

What is the total cooking time, including prep time?

Prep Time : _______________

Cook Time : _______________

Servings   : _______________

Ingredients:

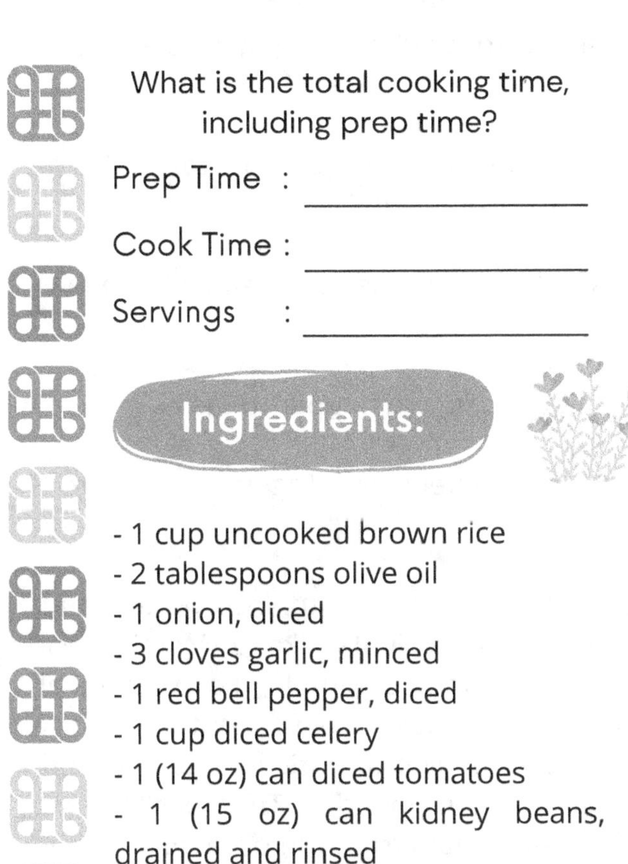

- 1 cup uncooked brown rice
- 2 tablespoons olive oil
- 1 onion, diced
- 3 cloves garlic, minced
- 1 red bell pepper, diced
- 1 cup diced celery
- 1 (14 oz) can diced tomatoes
- 1 (15 oz) can kidney beans, drained and rinsed
- 1 (15 oz) can black beans, drained and rinsed
- 2 cups vegetable broth
- 1 teaspoon smoked paprika
- 1 teaspoon dried thyme
- 1 teaspoon dried oregano
- 1/2 teaspoon cayenne pepper (optional, for heat)
- Salt and pepper to taste
- Chopped green onions for garnish (optional)

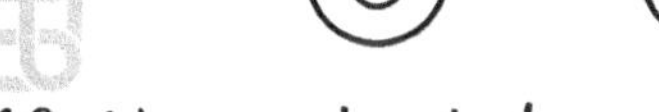

Is the recipe easy to follow?

1. Cook the brown rice according to package instructions. Set aside.

2. In a large pot or Dutch oven, heat the olive oil over medium heat. Add the onion and sauté for 5 minutes until translucent.

3. Add the garlic, bell pepper, and celery. Sauté for 3-4 minutes until the vegetables are tender.

4. Stir in the diced tomatoes, kidney beans, black beans, vegetable broth, smoked paprika, thyme, oregano, and cayenne (if using). Bring the mixture to a simmer.

5. Reduce heat to low and let the jambalaya simmer for 15-20 minutes, stirring occasionally, until the flavors have melded and the sauce has thickened slightly.

6. Stir in the cooked brown rice and season with salt and pepper to taste.

7. Serve hot, garnished with chopped green onions if desired.

This vegan jambalaya is packed with anti-inflammatory ingredients like bell peppers, celery, beans, and brown rice. The spices and herbs also provide additional anti-inflammatory benefits. It's a hearty, flavorful dish that can be a great option for seniors looking to incorporate more plant-based, anti-inflammatory foods into their diet.

110. Vegan Jambalaya with Brown Rice

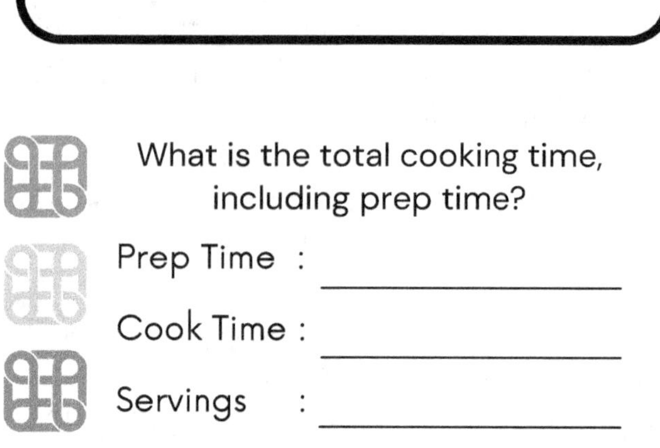

What are the critical points in the recipe (e.g., temperature control, timing)?

What is the total cooking time, including prep time?

Prep Time : _______________

Cook Time : _______________

Servings   : _______________

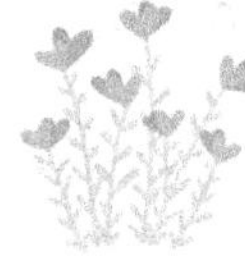

Ingredients:

- 3-4 medium zucchinis, spiralized or julienned into noodles
- 1/2 cup basil pesto (store-bought or homemade)
- 1/4 cup cherry tomatoes, halved
- 2 tablespoons toasted pine nuts
- 1 tablespoon grated Parmesan cheese (optional)
- Salt and pepper to taste

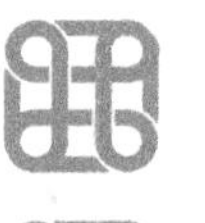
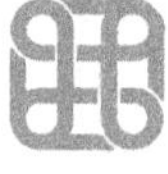
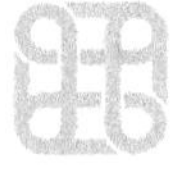
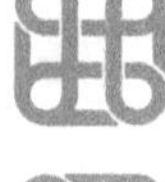
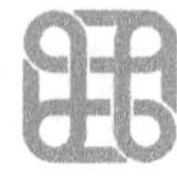

Is the recipe easy to follow?

111. Zucchini Noodles with Pesto

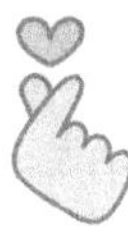

Procedure:

1. Prepare the zucchini noodles using a spiralizer, julienne peeler, or mandoline slicer. Set aside.

2. In a large bowl, toss the zucchini noodles with the basil pesto until the noodles are evenly coated.

3. Add the cherry tomatoes and toasted pine nuts. Gently mix to combine.

4. If desired, sprinkle the Parmesan cheese over the top.

5. Season with salt and pepper to taste.

6. Serve immediately, or refrigerate for up to 3 days.

This dish is a great way to incorporate anti-inflammatory ingredients like zucchini, basil, and pine nuts into a simple, flavorful meal. Zucchini is a low-calorie, nutrient-dense vegetable that is high in antioxidants and anti-inflammatory compounds. The basil pesto provides healthy fats from the olive oil and pine nuts, which can also help reduce inflammation.

This dish is easy to prepare, light, and refreshing, making it a great option for seniors looking for a nutritious and anti-inflammatory meal. You can also add grilled chicken or shrimp for additional protein if desired.

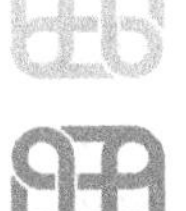

What is the total cooking time, including prep time?

Prep Time : ___________________

Cook Time : ___________________

Servings : ___________________

Ingredients:

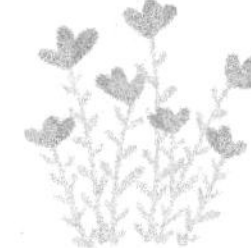

- 1 head of cauliflower, riced (about 4 cups riced cauliflower)
- 2 tablespoons olive oil
- 1 onion, diced
- 3 cloves garlic, minced
- 1 cup mixed frozen vegetables (such as peas, carrots, corn)
- 2 eggs, lightly beaten
- 2 tablespoons low-sodium soy sauce or tamari
- 1 teaspoon sesame oil
- Salt and pepper to taste
- Chopped green onions for garnish (optional)

Is the recipe easy to follow?

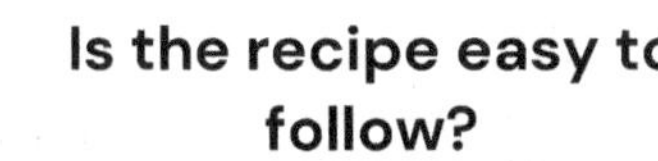

112. Cauliflower Fried Rice with Vegetables

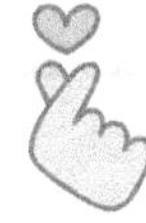

Procedure:

1. In a food processor, pulse the cauliflower florets until they resemble rice-sized pieces. Set aside.

2. In a large skillet or wok, heat the olive oil over medium-high heat. Add the onion and sauté for 3-4 minutes until translucent.

3. Add the garlic and sauté for 1 minute until fragrant.

4. Add the riced cauliflower and frozen vegetables to the skillet. Sauté for 5-7 minutes, stirring frequently, until the cauliflower is tender.

5. Push the cauliflower mixture to the side of the pan. Pour the beaten eggs into the empty side and scramble them, then mix them into the cauliflower mixture.

6. Stir in the soy sauce and sesame oil. Season with salt and pepper to taste.

7. Serve hot, garnished with chopped green onions if desired.

This cauliflower fried rice is a great alternative to traditional fried rice, providing a boost of anti-inflammatory nutrients from the cauliflower, vegetables, and healthy fats from the olive and sesame oils. The eggs also add protein to help keep seniors feeling full and satisfied.

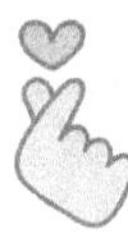

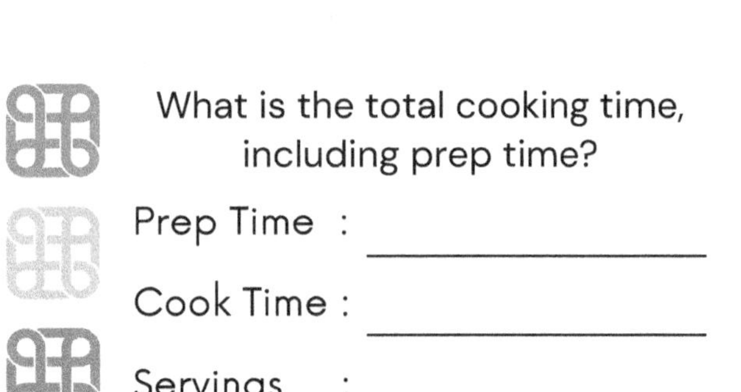

What is the total cooking time, including prep time?

Prep Time : ________________

Cook Time : ________________

Servings   : ________________

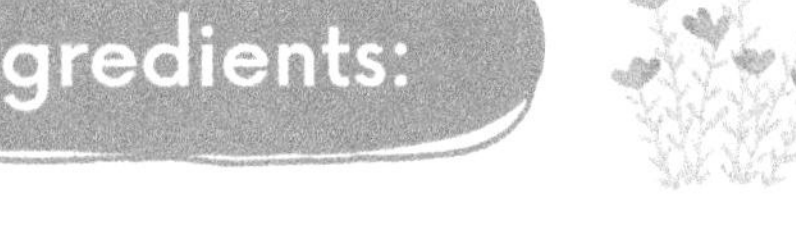

Ingredients:

- 1 medium spaghetti squash, halved lengthwise and seeds removed
- 2 tablespoons olive oil
- 1 onion, diced
- 3 cloves garlic, minced
- 1 (28 oz) can diced tomatoes
- 2 tablespoons tomato paste
- 1 teaspoon dried oregano
- 1/2 teaspoon dried basil
- Salt and pepper to taste
- Grated Parmesan cheese (optional)
- Chopped fresh basil for garnish (optional)

Is the recipe easy to follow?

113. Spaghetti Squash with Tomato Sauce

1. Preheat the oven to 400°F. Place the spaghetti squash halves cut-side down on a baking sheet. Bake for 40-50 minutes, until the squash is tender and easily shreds with a fork.

2. While the squash is baking, heat the olive oil in a large skillet over medium heat. Add the onion and sauté for 5-7 minutes until translucent.

3. Add the garlic and sauté for 1 minute until fragrant.

4. Stir in the diced tomatoes, tomato paste, oregano, and basil. Bring the sauce to a simmer and let it cook for 10-15 minutes, stirring occasionally, until thickened.

5. Season the tomato sauce with salt and pepper to taste.

6. Once the spaghetti squash is cooked, use a fork to shred the flesh into spaghetti-like strands.

7. Serve the spaghetti squash noodles topped with the tomato sauce. Garnish with grated Parmesan cheese and chopped fresh basil, if desired.

This dish is a great way to incorporate anti-inflammatory ingredients like spaghetti squash, tomatoes, and olive oil into a simple, flavorful meal. Spaghetti squash is a low-calorie, nutrient-dense vegetable that is high in antioxidants and anti-inflammatory compounds. The tomato sauce provides additional anti-inflammatory benefits from the lycopene in the tomatoes.

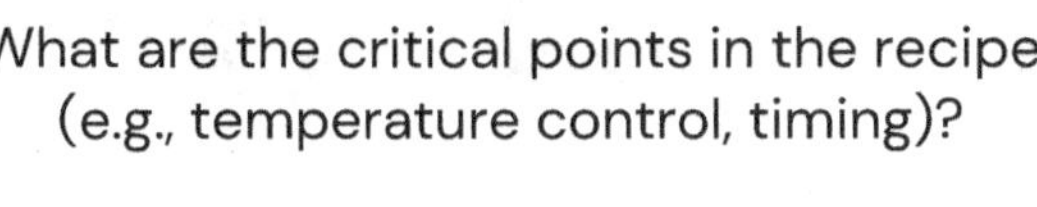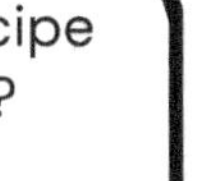

What are the critical points in the recipe (e.g., temperature control, timing)?

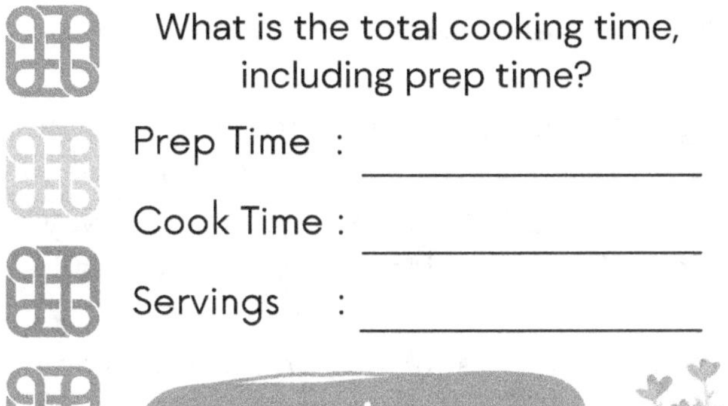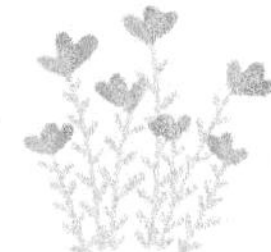

What is the total cooking time, including prep time?

Prep Time : _______________

Cook Time : _______________

Servings   : _______________

Ingredients:

- 4 bell peppers (any color), halved lengthwise and seeds removed
- 1 cup cooked brown or green lentils
- 1 cup cooked brown rice
- 1 onion, diced
- 3 cloves garlic, minced
- 1 (14 oz) can diced tomatoes
- 1 teaspoon dried oregano
- 1 teaspoon dried basil
- 1/4 teaspoon red pepper flakes (optional)
- Salt and pepper to taste
- 1/2 cup shredded mozzarella cheese (optional)

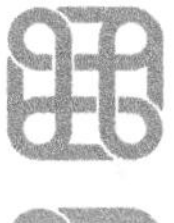

Is the recipe easy to follow?

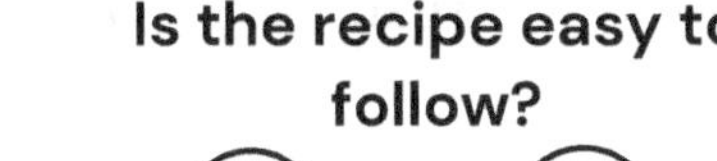

114. Stuffed Bell Peppers with Lentils

Procedure:

1. Preheat the oven to 375°F.

2. Place the bell pepper halves in a baking dish and set aside.

3. In a large skillet, sauté the onion in a bit of olive oil over medium heat for 5-7 minutes until translucent.

4. Add the garlic and sauté for 1 minute until fragrant.

5. Stir in the cooked lentils, brown rice, diced tomatoes, oregano, basil, and red pepper flakes (if using). Season with salt and pepper to taste.

6. Spoon the lentil-rice mixture into the bell pepper halves, packing it in gently.

7. If using, sprinkle the shredded mozzarella cheese over the top of the stuffed peppers.

8. Bake for 25-30 minutes, or until the peppers are tender and the filling is hot.

9. Serve the stuffed peppers warm.

This dish is a great way to incorporate anti-inflammatory ingredients like bell peppers, lentils, and tomatoes into a satisfying meal. Bell peppers are rich in vitamins and antioxidants, while lentils provide plant-based protein and fiber. The tomatoes add lycopene, an anti-inflammatory compound.

The combination of the nutrient-dense vegetables, plant-based protein, and healthy carbohydrates makes this a well-balanced and anti-inflammatory option for seniors. You can also customize the filling with additional herbs, spices, or vegetables to suit your taste preferences.

What are the critical points in the recipe (e.g., temperature control, timing)?

What is the total cooking time, including prep time?

Prep Time : _______________

Cook Time : _______________

Servings   : _______________

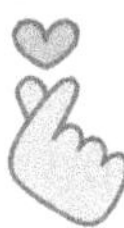

Ingredients:

Cashew Cheese:
- 1 cup raw cashews, soaked in water for at least 4 hours or overnight
- 1/4 cup water
- 2 tablespoons lemon juice
- 1 garlic clove
- 1/2 teaspoon salt

Lasagna:
- 2 medium eggplants, sliced lengthwise into 1/4-inch thick slices
- 2 tablespoons olive oil
- 1 onion, diced
- 3 cloves garlic, minced
- 1 (28 oz) can diced tomatoes
- 2 tablespoons tomato paste
- 1 teaspoon dried oregano
- 1/2 teaspoon dried basil
- Salt and pepper to taste
- Fresh basil leaves for garnish (optional)

115. Eggplant Lasagna with Cashew Cheese

Procedure:

1. Make the cashew cheese: Drain and rinse the soaked cashews. Add them to a high-speed blender or food processor along with the water, lemon juice, garlic, and salt. Blend until smooth and creamy. Set aside.

2. Preheat the oven to 375°F.

3. Arrange the eggplant slices in a single layer on a baking sheet. Brush both sides with olive oil. Bake for 15-20 minutes, flipping halfway, until the eggplant is tender and lightly browned.

4. In a large skillet, sauté the onion in a bit of olive oil over medium heat for 5-7 minutes until translucent. Add the garlic and sauté for 1 minute.

5. Stir in the diced tomatoes, tomato paste, oregano, and basil. Season with salt and pepper to taste. Simmer the sauce for 10-15 minutes, stirring occasionally, until thickened.

6. Assemble the lasagna: Spread a thin layer of the tomato sauce in the bottom of a baking dish. Arrange a layer of the roasted eggplant slices over the sauce. Spread a layer of the cashew cheese over the eggplant. Repeat the layers of sauce, eggplant, and cashew cheese until all the ingredients are used up, ending with the cashew cheese.

7. Bake the lasagna for 30-35 minutes, until the top is lightly browned and the filling is bubbly.

8. Let the lasagna cool for 10-15 minutes before serving. Garnish with fresh basil leaves, if desired.

Thank you for exploring the **"Vegan Anti-Inflammatory Cookbook for Seniors: 110+ Vegan Recipes for Seniors to Naturally Reduce Inflammation and Promote Health."** We hope this collection of recipes has inspired you to embrace the benefits of a plant-based, anti-inflammatory diet and made it easy and enjoyable to incorporate these nutritious meals into your daily routine.

Embracing a Healthier Lifestyle

Throughout this cookbook, you've discovered that eating healthfully doesn't have to be complicated or time-consuming. By focusing on simple, delicious vegan recipes, you can effectively reduce inflammation and support your overall health and well-being. The recipes provided have shown that nutritious meals can also be flavorful and satisfying, making it easier to maintain a healthy lifestyle.

Enhancing Wellness

By choosing anti-inflammatory foods, you're taking a proactive step towards improving your health. Whether you're managing a chronic condition or simply seeking to enhance your vitality, the recipes and tips in this cookbook offer a practical and enjoyable way to support your body's natural healing processes and promote longevity.

Continuing Your Culinary Journey

As you continue your journey towards better health, remember that the principles you've learned here can be applied to countless other recipes and cooking techniques. Experiment with new ingredients, explore different flavor combinations, and personalize the recipes to suit your tastes and dietary needs. The key is to keep it simple, nutritious, and enjoyable.

Celebrating Health and Flavor

Cooking and eating should be experiences that bring joy and satisfaction. We hope that the "Vegan Anti-Inflammatory Cookbook for Seniors" has helped you discover new favorite meals and a deeper appreciation for the benefits of anti-inflammatory foods. By embracing these recipes, you're not only nourishing your body but also enhancing your quality of life.

Thank you for choosing this cookbook and investing in your health. We hope that the recipes and knowledge shared here will continue to benefit you and your loved ones for years to come. Here's to a life filled with delicious meals, reduced inflammation, and vibrant health.

Happy cooking and good health!